Large-Scale Brain Systems
and Neuropsychological Testin

Leonard F. Koziol • Paul Beljan
Kate Bree • John Mather • Lauren Barker

Large-Scale Brain Systems and Neuropsychological Testing

An Effort to Move Forward

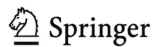 Springer

Leonard F. Koziol
Park Ridge, IL, USA

Kate Bree
Phoenix, AZ, USA

Lauren Barker
Chicago, IL, USA

Paul Beljan
Scottsdale, AZ, USA

John Mather
Mesa, AZ, USA

ISBN 978-3-319-80300-5   ISBN 978-3-319-28222-0   (eBook)
DOI 10.1007/978-3-319-28222-0

Printed on acid-free paper

This Springer imprint is published by Springer Nature
The registered company is Springer International Publishing AG Switzerland

To Sabrina,
Thank you for teaching me more about life than
you could ever imagine. I will always remember
you as my very special person.

Leonard F. Koziol

For my dear Jothi—everything fell into place
when I met you.

Paul Beljan

To the patients who inspired this work and to my
husband and family who supported me in
completing it. A special thanks to my mother,
Joan Wilson, M.D., for providing invaluable
consultation on prenatal factors in brain
development.

Kate Bree

To Kailea and Addison,
Your father helped to author a book about the
brain...even though I know I have convinced you
I do not have one. Thanks for making me love
and laugh!

John Mather

To Bryan, whose unconditional love and support
continues to help me become the best person and
practitioner I can be, and to Daisy, who shows
me every day that lifelong friends come in all
shapes and forms.

Lauren Barker

Authorship Statement
*The ordering of authorship does not imply
significance of contribution or level
of participation. All authors contributed
significant time, effort, and thought
to this work.*

∫

Introduction

Many practitioners are taught neuropsychology from a cortico-centric viewpoint, understanding the cortex as the primary driver of behavior. Although many of Luria's hypotheses about specific brain-behavior relationships have not withstood the test of time, at least two general neuropsychological ideas were critical to the way he seemed to organize his thinking. He recognized the role of subcortical processes in cognition and behavior, and he understood that how a behavior was performed informed the interpretation of brain-behavior relationships. Others before him, such as Goldstein and Jackson, had similar ideas [1, 2], but without a doubt, Lurian neuropsychology did influence western clinical neuropsychology, primarily through the development and introduction of a standardized, norm-based methodology for clinical application [3]. Focusing upon the qualitative features of behavior was never central to western neuropsychology, and in general, the neocortex was always considered the primary driver of cognition. Subcortical structures such as the basal ganglia and cerebellum were primarily considered coprocessors of movement. In addition, much of neuropsychology was organized around a fixed hemispheric view of the lateralization of brain function; the left hemisphere was considered dominant for language, and the right hemisphere was assigned a secondary role in "visuospatial" information processing and analysis, perhaps a carry-over from the era of Broca and Wernicke. Current neuroscience has taught us that the way in which behavior is organized within the brain is not so simple, but clinical neuropsychology seems to have adhered to a simple verbal-nonverbal hemispheric lateralization dichotomy. For example, testing methodologies were developed to localize brain pathology within the left or right hemispheres or perhaps the anterior and/or posterior hemispheres. Although our summary is oversimplified, little, if any, attention was paid to subcortical structures or processes in the understanding of cognition and the development of assessment measures.

From a simple, common sense point of view, this seems somewhat ironic, as it is well accepted that the physical development of the brain occurs from the "bottom-up" and from "inside to outside." In neuropsychological and pathophysiological nomenclature, the brain develops from proximal to distal brain regions. Nevertheless, the focus has always been placed upon the human cortex with respect to understanding cognition and the interpretation of neuropsychological test results. We follow an alternative viewpoint, but not quite the opposite, as has been described in *ADHD as a Model of Brain-Behavior Relationships* and *The Myth of Executive Functioning*, published by Springer in 2013 and 2014, respectively. For us, there is unequivocal evidence that the basal ganglia serve as a cognitive and behavioral selection mechanism [4], while the cerebellum serves as a coprocessor of the cerebral cortex, working together with it as an ensemble! [5]. We are not exactly boldly proposing a 180° turn by stating clinical neuropsychology and its assessment methods have it all wrong! Instead, we are saying that clinical neuropsychology's understanding of cognition, and behavior, is incomplete. However, this lack of completeness overlooks so much of the integrated brain that test results generate numerous interpretative errors. This greatly limits the utility of neuropsychological evaluations, and within today's healthcare and academic environments, these limitations threaten the survival of the profession.

Perhaps this "cortex is king" thinking was arguably appropriate many years ago, when neuropsychology was literally in its infancy and when brain-behavior relationships were first being studied and measured. Structure and function relationships were often derived from the identification of cortical lesions during postmortem examination and/or inferred from lesion studies with animals. In our opinion, these ways of learning about brain function also led to a *static* view of cognition [6]. However, as the varying fields of the neurosciences have advanced, significant progress has been made in understanding brain-behavior relationships. For one, neuroimaging allows neurologists and neuropsychologists to view brain structures and functioning in real time, rather than relying on postmortem findings and correlating them with behaviors during life. And in this regard, we can understand cognition and adaptation as *dynamically changing* processes. Neuropsychological assessment measures currently view much of cognition as static, while tests are interpreted within a serial-ordering processing paradigm. Within this paradigm, first we perceive; then we think; and finally we respond. But do cognition, behavior, and adaptation really work that way? As described in the first two volumes of this series, people are constantly thinking and behaving in an interactive way. Cognition, behavior, and pathologies need to be understood within an interpretive paradigm that emphasizes *ongoing sensory-motor interaction and adaptation.* So neuropsychology needs to address the question of how tests based upon a static view of cognition might be interpreted within an interactive paradigm. And this should lead to the question of how to develop methodologies and tests that allow us to achieve that level of understanding within clinical settings. We hope this book represents at least a small step in facing these interpretive challenges.

In an attempt to standardize neuropsychological assessment data and interpretative outcomes, the field has relied upon organizing and interpreting data within the parameters of the normally distributed bell-shaped curve; we are at a total loss in trying to explain why this has occurred since numerous neurocognitive skills and behaviors are skewed in their distribution. Therefore, interpretation of neuropsychological assessment results based upon the bell-shaped curve is often inappropriate and fails to consider pathognomonic signs and the fact that neuropsychological deficits do not conform to a normally distributed bell-shaped curve. Considering all data as if they were normally distributed yields scores that can provide a false sense of security as test results are simply described categorically, as average, low average, above average, etc. However, this seemingly ancient statistical methodology has potentially left an ocean of misdiagnosed and undiagnosed patients in its wake. What do these overarching, umbrella terms really mean? What diagnosis, or what symptoms, do these terms identify?

The Halstead-Reitan neuropsychological test battery was perhaps the first collection of organized neuropsychological tasks that assessed a variety of seemingly different cognitive, sensory, and motor functions. While certain tasks within the battery might have followed the normal distribution of a bell-shaped curve, some tests were interpreted in terms of "raw scores," without performing any statistical transformations whatsoever. Raw score cutoff points were developed for many tasks, and then one performance was compared to a different relevant task score. Other tasks were clearly of pathognomonic significance. So a variety of interpretative methodologies grew out of the HRB approach. These facts make it even more difficult to understand why it seems as though most of today's neuropsychological testing employs the "standard score" and/or "normal distribution" interpretative approach. The HRB interpretative methodologies, or "levels of inference," worked! Why, and how, did they vanish in favor of an uninformative statistical approach? Perhaps it was because Reitan's tests were never revised; the tests themselves were bulky and very difficult to transport; however, as these tests became less and less popular, neuropsychology seemed to throw out the baby with the bath water. The clinical beauty of the HRB, in our opinion, had little or nothing to do with test content. Instead, it was the methodology and the levels of clinical inference that were the most important contributions to clinical neuropsychology. Virtually any number of tests could have been interpreted within the inferential methodology; very large, cumbersome amounts of data could have been structured, organized, and interpreted within that methodological framework. As the HRB decreased in clinical application, the most significant contribution to neuropsychology, the interpretative framework, was abandoned. Throughout this volume, we attempt to restore those levels of inferential analysis because that framework is extremely valuable for today's neuroscience.

Early Studies in Clinical Neuropsychology

Halstead and Reitan essentially viewed the brain as composed of four separate quadrants—the left and right hemispheres and the anterior and posterior regions of the brain [7]. Observable lines of neuroanatomic demarcation were applied to divide the brain into these regions, resulting in the division of the brain into the left frontal lobe, the right frontal lobe, the left posterior cortical lobes (i.e., the temporal, parietal, and occipital lobes), and the right posterior cortical lobes [7]. Therefore, Hallstead and Reitan interpreted neuropsychological results based upon the believed functions of these quadrants [7]. And these functional brain regions were considered static and not representative of brain interactions.

While the field was in its infancy, Broca and Wernicke discovered that, for the majority of humans, language resides solely in the left hemisphere; therefore, the left hemisphere became known as the dominant hemisphere of the cerebral cortex [6]. The right hemisphere became a brain region of less importance; however, today we know that nothing could be further from the truth [8]. While it was once believed that the left hemisphere was the sole processor of language-related information and the right hemisphere processed the so-called nonverbal information, this fixed hemispheric assignment is now unequivocally known to be untrue. It should be widely accepted today that the left hemisphere is not irrelevant to nonverbal functions nor is the right hemisphere irrelevant to verbal functions. The initial dichotomy between hemispheric functions should be accepted as a universal falsehood, although based upon our early understanding of brain-behavior relationships, the assumptions represented seemingly reasonable starting points for examining brain-behavior relationships. This principle became tradition. It became a habitual way of thinking—and habits are hard to break.

As an aside, what is nonverbal function/cognition? Can anything truly be nonverbal once language has developed? For example, one cannot think of or visualize the color orange without thinking of the word *orange* [9]. Functional magnetic resonance imaging (fMRI) studies show how language tracts are recruited when one is learning to play a musical instrument, but the same tracts are not recruited when the skill is habituated [10]. Language is the function that links human thinking with action [11]. Although one may claim that music is a language because it evokes emotion, one certainly cannot write a symphony that teaches algebra to a math student.

Much as the concept of nonverbal skills has been retained as a truism despite evidence to the contrary, clinical neuropsychology has not really progressed past many early assumptions regarding brain-behavior relationships. This is extremely unfortunate because present biases potentially result in misleading diagnostic conclusions. Despite their oversimplified view of brain structure and function, Hallstead's and Reitan's work has provided a way of quantifying brain functions so that studies of various types of brain pathologies could be duplicated from one laboratory to another and so that consistent findings could be replicated. The positive aspect of this approach represented the emphasis upon quantification; however, the negative aspect of this methodology evolved into the idea that qualitative observations are less important than quantifiable evaluation outcomes.

Unlike Halstead and Reitan, Luria emphasized the qualitative approach of interpreting brain functioning. Luria actually believed that subcortical regions were paramount with respect to brain-behavior relationships, although the methodologies that he emphasized were never subject to statistical investigation [12]. When Lurian methodologies were introduced to and eventually integrated into western neuropsychology, the immediate emphasis was placed upon quantification. Something was lost in the translation, and that "something" was an important contribution toward understanding brain-behavior relationships. All behavior is purposeful [13]. The primary goal inherent in the very definition of neuropsychology is determining how an individual brain functions, but that notion somehow got lost.

Contemporary neuropsychology has the benefit of quickly advancing neurotechnology—technology that was not available to guide Luria or Hallstead and Reitan in developing neurocognitive theories and testing methodologies. Admittedly this introduction provides a gross oversimplification; however, the authors hope the points being made remain clear. Neuroscience has made significant advancements over the past several decades, yet clinical neuropsychology has remained steadfast in the utilization of quantifiable, cortico-centric neuropsychological test construction and interpretation. Our intent in writing this introduction was to be just that simple–nothing more, nothing less. A comprehensive approach to studying how the field of neuropsychology or its assessment measures evolved Or developed was never the goal. The purpose of this oversimplification is to present the reader with the clear, obvious, and dramatic dichotomy between the profound advancements in neuroimaging and the profound steadfastness of clinical neuropsychology in its adherence to outdated theories, assessment methods, and interpretations. Although tradition and habit are hard to break, it is time for the field to question the status quo. Realizing, accepting, and applying the idea that something that may no longer be the most salient explanation and/or the most effective methodology for assessment and interpretation are fundamental to any scientific inquiry. Our goal is to violate well-entrenched theories and practices and to compel those in the field of neuropsychology to take a step back for a moment to analyze contemporary notions of neuropsychological assessment and interpretation. In this way, we are continuing with the intentions for ADHD as a Model of Brain-Behavior Relationships and The Myth of Executive Functioning [14, 15].

In 2009, Koziol and Budding, in a book titled *Subcortical Structures and Cognition: Implications for Neuropsychological Assessment* [16], emphasized several critical points. The book provided a summary of the role of subcortical structures in what might be termed higher-level thought processes. It was demonstrated that current neuropsychological tests are poor at brain localization (so-called lesion hunting) because brain function is not purely neocortical and because subcortical structures are often overlooked in test interpretation. It was conclusively demonstrated that few new methodologies have been proposed in clinical neuropsychology, despite significant advances in other branches of clinical neuroscience. The reader was hopefully left with the idea that clinical neuropsychology lags far behind the times when the field is compared to the "hard" neurosciences which study brain-behavior relationships and brain-behavior pathologies. That monograph was, and remains, a tough controversial nut to crack. Similarly, it is hard to give up ideas of fixed hemispheric assignment of functions. However, without expanding our horizons by including dynamic brain interactions in interpreting task performance, and without considering *brain network* functions, it is impossible for clinical neuropsychology to maintain, or perhaps establish, any semblance of clinical usefulness.

From Movement to Thought

Borrowing from Schmahmann and a host of others [17], Koziol and Budding [16] were arguably the first two neuropsychologist-authors who discussed the non-motor functions of the basal ganglia and the cerebellum in a systematic fashion; however, nothing they presented was "new." In fact, nothing they presented was original or innovative, yet these ideas readily emerged from a thorough, comprehensive review of research within various fields of the neurosciences. Despite the fact that the viewpoint and conclusions were not novel at the time, it seems the field of clinical neuropsychology has yet to accept the incredibly important and evident role of the basal ganglia and cerebellum in brain-behavior relationships. Perhaps this demonstrates how slowly fields change and grow; research-based data are not quickly applied within certain clinical settings. Through their work, Koziol and Budding clearly and convincingly concluded that the basal ganglia play a significant role in a variety of behaviors and that the cerebellum similarly plays a critical adaptive role in human functioning, regardless of whether or not those functions were motor or cognitive. Prior to their writing there was no systematic review of how the basal ganglia and the cerebellum contribute to higher-level cognitive functions that do not include a motor component, yet it became clear that the brain functions as an integrated, well-orchestrated unit that inseparably couples cognition with action/motor output. Numerous case presentations demonstrated how certain patterns of neuropsychological test results mimicked basal ganglia and/or cerebellar pathologies. Novel ways of applying currently available neuropsychological tests to understanding basal ganglia and cerebellar functioning/pathology were offered. They basically returned to variations of Reitan's methods of inferential analysis to illustrate how tasks used as "probes" in neuropsychological experimental studies could be integrated into clinical practice/assessment in order to provide a better understanding of patients.

In 2013, Koziol, Budding, and Chidekel authored *ADHD as a Model of Brain-Behavior Relationships* [14]. In that concise volume, ADHD was examined as the cognitive, emotional, and behavioral product of the interaction of neocortical, basal ganglia, and cerebellar processes. It was proposed that ADHD, or any other pathology, could be similarly considered as a model for understanding brain-behavior relationships, because the vertebrate brain has been consistent in its organization for over 500 million years of evolution, while all critical brain functions have been preserved throughout the course of phylogeny [6]. Similarly, it was again emphasized that neuropsychology was in a position of taking experimental neuroscientific test findings and using those exact same paradigms in order to identify better methodologies to understand and assess human brain-behavior relationships [14]. Therefore, clinical neuropsychology would align more directly and keep pace with contemporary neuroscience. More importantly, the issues of differential diagnosis, symptom identification, and patient treatment would be enhanced.

In 2014, Koziol published *The Myth of Executive Functioning: Missing Elements in Conceptualization, Evaluation, and Assessment* [15]. This succinct monograph redefined the concept of executive functioning cognitive processes. Executive functions were presented as a neurobiologically situated expansion of the cortico-basal ganglia and the cerebro-cerebellar circuitry systems. In a persuasive empirically informed argument, the term "executive functioning" was banished in favor of understanding all behavior as the product of a cognitive control system. The emphasis was placed upon action control in order to achieve adaptive behavior. This always requires a coupling of perceptual/ideational-action (i.e., sensory-motor) in order to meet the challenges of constantly interacting with changing sensory-motor environments and demands. And not much of this behavior is under the mediation of thinking of which a person is consciously aware. Methods of examining cognitive control were offered, and once again, it was proposed that clinical neuropsychology was in need of modifying current test procedures and developing new tasks and/or evaluation paradigms to assess the issues of adaptation across the age span and across various pathologies. The argument was and remains appealing based upon its simplicity, its practicality, and its neurobiological consistency with the current neuroscience of large-scale brain systems and interactions with subcortical structures, as well as with its adherence to a model of overall cognitive control based upon current views of the brain as an anticipatory control mechanism. Subsequent writings [18–21] reemphasized that "cognitive" does not necessarily translate to "conscious awareness."

Alas, we propose the field of neuropsychology has stagnated of late in terms of understanding brain-behavior relationships. Simply put, as *The Myth of Executive Functioning* concluded, perhaps we are right back where we started in focusing upon cortico-centric ideas and interpretive methodologies that focus almost entirely on numerical, statistical, and quantifiable methods. No one is proposing that these traditional methodologies being used are unimportant or irrelevant. Nevertheless, it must be acknowledged that there is a striking absence of any new clinical methodologies that have resulted in a deeper and more precise understanding of human brain-behavior functioning. Furthermore, a distinction must be made between developing and applying a new methodology and constructing a new test.

The original works of Lezak [22] and Spreen and Strauss [23] are frequently updated as reviews of new neuropsychological tests are introduced into the commercial market. Many neuropsychologists naively use tests as if the specific name of the test had face validity, when to the contrary, it has been well documented that neuropsychological tests do not offer face validity. More often than not, these tests do not evaluate what they purport to measure! Many tests are atheoretical in organization and are not based upon the manner in which test/task behavior is organized within the human brain [24]. There might be a false sense of security that goes along with the concept of face validity, but there is no substitute for test interpretation based upon an understanding of functional neuroanatomy. Isn't neuropsychology defined as the study of brain-behavior relationships? In any other profession, a lack of understanding of what a test measures would be completely unacceptable. Fortunately for the general population, most medical tests are not named as if they could possibly be interpreted according to concepts of artificial face validity, so that an understanding of symptoms and the neurobiological processes that drive them must be grasped before making a clinical diagnosis and deciding upon the proper treatment/intervention. But why should clinical neuropsychology be any different? As Lezak [22], Kaplan [25], and others too numerous to mention have always stated, tests do not make a diagnosis; instead, clinicians do. In this regard, we ask the reader to pause and think about the tests you use and the underlying neuroanatomy that presumably drives the results of those tasks. If this model is not consistent with your way of thinking about test data interpretation, then take time for an extended pause to ponder about whether or not you want to read this volume. We assume the reader has a comprehensive understanding of the above references, although we will review certain concepts briefly and add to others for the purpose of maintaining clinical consistency.

This book was written with several purposes in mind. One purpose is to take the focus away from a cortico-centric understanding of behavior and to examine the roles subcortical structures play in supporting human behavior. Another purpose of this volume is to interpret case studies by using neuropsychological tests which are currently available and widely used, but in a slightly different way. The authors propose changes to existing methodology that would shed light on a much deeper understanding of brain-behavior relationships. In addition, the understanding that emerges is directly applicable to not only disorder identification but also to developing appropriate treatment strategies. That is, every pathological observation and inference lends itself to a recommendation. Finally, this book closes by demonstrating the continuing missing links in current neuropsychological assessment, in order to promote the ongoing need for the introduction of new assessments techniques. Along the way, qualitative observations are applied in order to modify quantitative data, in an attempt to demonstrate how the original quantification techniques might be coupled together with other data to enhance behavioral understanding. Finally, we hope to illustrate perhaps the biggest challenges faced by clinical neuropsychology—how can we shift our thinking in order to interpret existing tests within an *interactive, dynamic* behavioral paradigm, and how are we to employ these tests, or others, within the context of *brain networks* that change during the course of task performance?

It should be fully understood that we are not taking sole authorship or intellectual ownership for the material presented in this volume. The neocortex, basal ganglia, and cerebellum have been extensively studied by others. We are not self-appointed leaders in this field. Instead, we are standing on the shoulders of an enormous reference base, as illustrated in *ADHD as a Model of Brain-Behavior Relationships* and *The Myth of Executive Functioning*, to empirically inform the thinking that makes this volume possible. We are merely integrating the findings and ideas of others from a project that began in 2009 with the writing of *Subcortical Structures and Cognition: Implications for Neuropsychological Testing*. This volume is another building block to assist in bridging the gap between neuropsychology and neuroscientific fields for the purpose of better helping the populations we serve. We hope this work contributes to a better understanding of the cortex, the basal ganglia, and the cerebellum, in both health and disease.

References

1. Pow, S., & Stahnisch, F. W. (2014). Kurt Goldstein (1878–1965). *Journal of Neurology, 261*(5), 1049–1050. doi:10.1007/s00415-013-7020-1.
2. York, G. K., & Steinberg, D. A. (2006). An introduction to the life and work of John Hughlings Jackson with a catalogue raisonné of his writings. *Medical History Supplement, (26)*, 3–34.
3. Golden, C. J., Hammeke, T. A., & Purisch, A. D. (1978). Diagnostic validity of a standardized neuro-psychological battery derived from Luria's neuropsychological tests. *Journal of Consulting and Clinical Psychology, 46*, 1258–1265.
4. Hikosaka, O., & Isoda, M. (2010). Switching from automatic to controlled behavior: cortico-basal ganglia mechanisms. *Trends in Cognitive Sciences, 14*(4), 154–161.
5. Koziol, L. F., Budding, D., Andreasen, N., et al. (2014). Consensus paper: The Cerebellum's role in movement and cognition. *Cerebellum, 13*(1), 151–177.
6. Kolb, B., & Whishaw, I. Q. (2014). *An introduction to brain and behavior*. New York, NY: Worth.
7. Reitan, R. M. (1975). Human neuropsychology: Assessment of brain-behavior relationships. In P. McReynolds (Ed.), *Advances in psychological assessment* (Vol. 3, pp. 186–242). San Francisco, CA: Josey-Bass.
8. Trimble, M. R., & George, M. S. (2010). *Biological psychiatry* (3rd ed.). Chester, England: Wiley.
9. Winawer, J., Witthoft, N., Frank, M. C., Wu, L., Wade, A. R., & Boroditsky, L. (2007). Russian blues reveal effects of language on color discrimination. *Proceedings of the National Academy of Sciences, 104*(19), 7780–7785.
10. Schlaug, G. (2015). Musicians and music making as a model for the study of brain plasticity. *Progress in Brain Research, 217*, 37–55. doi:10.1016/bs.pbr.2014.11.020.
11. Cowley, S. J. (2014). Linguistic embodiment and verbal constraints: Human cognition and the scales of time. *Frontiers in Psychology, 5*, 1085. doi:10.3389/fpsyg.2014.01085.
12. Goldberg, E. (2001). *The executive brain* (1st ed.). New York, NY: Oxford University Press.
13. Wundt, W. (1907). *Principles of physiological psychology*. New York, NY: Macmillan.
14. Koziol, L. F., Budding, D. E., & Chidekel, D. (2013). *ADHD as a model of brain-behavior relationships*. New York, NY: Springer.
15. Koziol, L. F. (2014). *The myth of executive functioning: Missing elements in conceptualization, evaluation, and assessment*. New York, NY: Springer.
16. Koziol, L. F., & Budding, D. E. (2009). *Subcortical structures and cognition: Implications for neuropsychological assessment*. New York, NY: Springer.
17. Schmahmann, J. D. (1996). From movement to thought: Anatomic substrates of the cerebellar contribution to cognitive processing. *Human Brain Mapping, 4*, 174–198.
18. Koziol, L. F., Barker, L. A., Joyce, A. W., & Hrin, S. (2014). Structure and function of large-scale brain systems. *Applied Neuropsychology Child, 3*(4), 236–244.
19. Koziol, L. F., Barker, L. A., Joyce, A. W., & Hrin, S. (2014). The small-world organization of large-scale brain systems and relationships with subcortical structures. *Applied Neuropsychology Child, 3*(4), 245–252.
20. Koziol, L. F., Barker, L. A., Joyce, A. W., & Hrin, S. (2014). Large-scale brain systems and subcortical relationships: The vertically organized brain. *Applied Neuropsychology Child, 3*(4), 253–263.

21. Koziol, L. F., Barker, L. A., Hrin, S., & Joyce, A. W. (2014). Large-scale brain systems and subcortical relationships: Practical applications. *Applied Neuropsychology Child, 3*(4), 264–273.
22. Lezak, M. D., Howieson, D. B., Bigler, E. D., & Tranel, D. (2012). *Neuropsychological assessment* (5th ed.). New York, NY: Oxford University Press.
23. Strauss, E., Sherman, E. M. S., Spreen, O., & Spreen, O. (2006). *A compendium of neuropsychological tests: Administration, norms, and commentary.* Oxford, England: Oxford University Press.
24. Haynes, S. N., Richard, D. C. S., & Kubany, E. S. (1995). Content validity in psychological assessment: A functional approach to concepts and methods. *Psychological Assessment, 7*(3), 238–247.
25. Delis, D. (2010). Edith Kaplan (1924–2009). *American Psychologist, 65*(2), 127–128.

Contents

1 Basic Principles: Behavioral History and What It Means 1
Risk Factors, Information Integration, Over
and Under Using Data, and Report Phraseology 2
Developmental History and the Traditional Training Paradigm 4
Case 1 5
Apgar Scores: How Are They Useful? 10
A Selective Review of Basic Developmental "At Risk" Factors 10
Premature Birth 11
Feeding, Language, and Reward 12
Hyperbilirubinemia 14
Prenatal Reflexes: Why Are They Important? 15
The Progression from Sitting to Crawling to Walking:
Why Is This Important? 16
Additional Case Presentations 20
Case 2: An Erroneous and Misleading History 20
Case 3 22
Discussion 22
References 23

2 Methods of Neuropsychological Test Interpretation 27
Introduction 27
Additional Introductory Issues: Assumptions, Facts, and Biases 28
Collecting Clinical Data: Defining the Problems 31
Case 4: Timmy 34
The Quantification of Behavior 36
Levels of Inference in Neuropsychological Test Interpretation 37
The Level of Performance 38
Pattern Analysis 39
Pathognomonic Signs 40

The Analysis of Sensory and Motor Data 41
Interim Summary 44
Challenges for Neuropsychology 45
References 47

3   The Normal Distribution of the Bell-Shaped Curve 49
The Normal Distribution 50
Limitations of Standard Normal Distributions 52
Application and Misapplication of Statistical Processes 54
Chance Variation and Statistical Versus Clinical Significance 56
More About Statistical Conversions Versus Normal Distributions 58
References 60

4   Beyond the Bell-Shaped Curve 63
Intra-individual and Other Test Score Comparisons 63
The Medial Temporal Lobe Memory System 65
Interim Conclusions 71
More About Test Pattern Analysis 71
Summary 76
References 76

5   The Interpretive Significance of Pathognomonic Signs 79
False Positive and False Negative Errors 82
Pathognomonic Signs in Neuro-Developmental Disorders 83
Continuous Performance Tests, Stop Signal Tasks,
and Go-No Go Paradigms: Unfortunate Misunderstandings
and the Controversy 84
Case 5 89
Case 6 90
Reading and Spelling: Predictive Observations
and Pathognomonic Signs of Disorder 91
References 96

**6   Tradition and Innovation: Making the Neuropsychological
Evaluation a More Powerful Tool** 101
Practice Effect: What Is It and Should It Always Be Avoided? 103
Case 7 109
Perception/Idea-Action Coupling 112
Case 8 114
Case 9: RCFT Evidence of Compromised Functioning
Within the VAN, DAN, FPN, AND SMN Systems 118
Case 10: "Everything that Counts Cannot Be Counted" 122
Summary 124
References 126

7 Summary... 129
"You Can't Teach an Old Dog New Tricks":
Where Did Clinical Neuropsychology Go Wrong?.................................... 129
References.. 134

Index.. 137

Chapter 1
Basic Principles: Behavioral History and What It Means

"Even a mistake may turn out to be the one thing necessary to a worthwhile achievement."

Henry Ford

"Never tell people how to do things. Tell them what to do and they will surprise you with their ingenuity."

George S. Patton

"Nothing pains some people more than having to think."

Martin Luther King, Jr.

This chapter is about obtaining history information. Every neuropsychologist knows how to do this aspect of the evaluation. The focus of this chapter is more specific. In this day and age, the histories we obtain need to be more detailed; we need to delve more deeply into a person's background if only because recent years have taught us much more about neurodevelopmental factors than we ever knew before. Nevertheless, our knowledge of development still remains in its infancy. Different professions are highly specialized, these professions such as Speech/Language pathology and Occupational Therapy use developmental data to guide their interventions, and in many cases, neuropsychologists could benefit from the knowledge of those professions but they are not exposed to it. Therefore, this chapter focuses upon an updated information database and information integration. It examines certain features of development that are not only important, but also should be woven into the summary of the patient's report. The summary not only specifies the findings, but also provides the opportunity to integrate information from the person's history in order to better understand the objective test results, and then, stating the appropriate evidence-based interventions. This is particularly important in cases of pediatric neuropsychological assessment when complicated neurodevelopmental data can often make the presenting problems easier to understand. Developmental history is frequently unknown or difficult to fully ascertain when evaluating an

© Springer International Publishing Switzerland 2016
L.F. Koziol et al., *Large-Scale Brain Systems and Neuropsychological Testing*,
DOI 10.1007/978-3-319-28222-0_1

adult. Typically, a parent or caretaker is involved and capable of providing relevant and necessary background information during almost every pediatric assessment. However, dependent upon the case and the family's status, sufficient developmental history data is sometimes unattainable.

Risk Factors, Information Integration, Over and Under Using Data, and Report Phraseology

This chapter is also about "risk factors." When we use the terms "risk factor" or "at risk," we are referring to any anomaly in an infant or child history that has been documented within the professional literature to increase the likelihood for experiencing a neurodevelopmental disorder. *All "at risk" factors are evidence-based.* We frequently observe that historical information obtained via interview is characterized by numerous neurodevelopmental risk factors. Sometimes, obvious "risk factors" are appropriately listed in the "background" section of the neuropsychological report. At other times, "at risk" factors are either under or over-interpreted. Whoever reads this chapter probably has observed this when reviewing a report written by another practitioner. The opportunity to read another clinician's report occurs most often when examining a child for a second opinion, or when asked to perform an assessment as a follow-up, after a certain period of time. Under these conditions, it might become apparent that the prior examiner either over or under-reported the significance of "at risk" factors in a child's history. For example, premature birth is one such important risk factor. The most common lesion and the most frequently occurring neurodevelopmental pathology observed in very premature birth is periventricular leukomalacia (PVL). However, we have observed reports in which an examiner identified severe cognitive pathology and attributed the chronic and significant cognitive deficits to PVL, but there was never any documentation in the record that PVL was identified. The observed cognitive deficits could easily have been a manifestation of the multiple other "at risk" factors documented within the child's history. This is a very valid "best guess" because PVL never occurs in isolation in cases of premature birth [1]. This conclusion would therefore represent an over-interpretation of a birth history, since that particular "at risk" factor was never identified within the history to begin with. An examiner assumed the presence of a risk factor and used an assumption to explain etiology. The patient's history, and test data, very frequently do not explain causality. This is true of almost every profession, and clinical neuropsychology is no different. The purpose of the assessment is not to determine causality; the purpose is to understand a child's capabilities, to identify symptoms, to develop treatment plans, but not to provide support for possible undocumented pathologies. Neuropsychologists attempt to identify symptoms and their known underpinnings whenever possible. Knowing about "risk factors" supports that purpose. But there is no specific pattern of test data that aligns only with PVL.

In a similar vein, we have observed cases in which moderately high bilirubin levels complicated the management of health problems of the infant, documented within the medical record, as well as initial difficulties in "latching-on" for early breast feeding. The neuropsychological report described notable symptoms of inattention and distractibility, as well as early onset language problems—disturbances in both articulation and grammar. The report correctly identified numerous symptoms, but lacked integration with known developmental risk factors. It would have been useful to integrate all these aspects of the history, especially since the "risk factors" were well documented, evidence-based, and align well with known identified relationships with ADHD-like symptoms as well as signs of possible Specific Language Impairment, or SLI [2–4]. In this case, integrating these "associations" would have been useful, particularly with respect to longer-term prognostic outcomes. Just as importantly, integrating this information can easily affect the choice of treatment modalities (E.To, personal communication, summer, 2015). This type of integration need not directly address causality. For example, the observed symptoms easily could have been driven by hereditary influences as well [5]. But since the data are documented, an integrative summary should include all the relevant factors, since this type of integration, with multiple conclusions, is an enriched, much more useful report that can be much more meaningful for treatment providers. As reviewed in *ADHD as a Model of Brain-Behavior Relationships* [28], hereditary phenotypes of ADHD might respond more easily to psychostimulant medication, but "acquired" cases of ADHD (perhaps a later manifestation of hyperbilirubinemia) might not demonstrate such a robust medication response. And an evaluator who believes they have a "litmus test" for untangling hereditary from acquired factors might not be aware of all the relevant variables; anyone who thinks they can predict which symptoms are hereditary in origin versus those behaviors that are acquired simply will have difficulties in defending that position. A conservative stance is best, and this incorporates two important attitudes; first, if any "at risk" factors can be interpreted in multiple ways, there is no foundation for an exact interpretation based upon any one particular variable; all the possibilities are to be reviewed; second, the purpose of the clinical neuropsychological interview and evaluation is again not to prove or disprove causality. In our experience, lawyers can attempt to "bait" clinicians by asking questions that are impossible to answer because too many etiological possibilities exist. In forensic cases, do not take the bait. In any event, the example we gave would be an illustration of the under-interpretation of history and behavioral data when the conclusion does not integrate all "known" or documented variables. Therefore, trying to integrate historic "at risk" factors with other evaluation data can be a "tricky" process. The best "cure" for these issues for writing cohesive and integrated reports is to rely upon objective, documented history data, knowing about the sequelae of "risk factors", and only then integrating the data to provide an enriched understanding of the child.

Finally, as a general rule, recommendations should be handled with extreme care while considering risk factors, test data, and behavioral observations. The neuropsychologist does not have the authority to write recommendations for the need for medications. Nor does he/she have the ability to order neuroimaging tests. This does not mean opinions about these recommendations cannot or should not be stated. In fact, it is mandatory to take an objective stance, documenting something like, "this child has the type of cognitive profile which is described in the literature as responsive to psychostimulant medication." This is an evidence-based statement, entirely different from stating, "in my opinion, a trial of a psychostimulant medication is indicated." It is very plausible that a patient's medical status, unknown to the neuropsychologist, contraindicates certain types of treatment options. Along similar lines, stating that "this patient might benefit from an MRI of the brain" is one issue; reporting that "further neurologic evaluation, including a brain imaging study, is indicated in view of the patient's signs of mild cognitive impairment", is quite a different statement. Specific recommendations like this one are outside the realm of neuropsychological evaluation. A report that states that "options such as these are a matter for medical decision making" is a completely different statement. In our opinion, it is important for practitioners to define the limits and scope of their profession, and the aforementioned recommendations can nevertheless be made by respecting the purview of other professions which in reality are responsible for the patient's care. The "bottom line" here is hopefully clear; *know your evidence-based risk factors, know how to define your limits, and apply them properly.*

Developmental History and the Traditional Training Paradigm

Birth complications are relatively common. In some cases, these complications require little attention. In other cases, a longer, more extensive hospitalization is necessary in order for the baby to stabilize. Obviously, the length of hospitalization does not predict specific long-term neuro-cognitive outcomes. However, a few additional points are in order. Any perinatal risk factor can be significant. From a neuropsychological perspective, the length of neonatal hospitalization does not define the significance of the risk factor, nor does this predict shorter or even longer-term neurodevelopmental outcomes. Sometimes a risk factor can seem so slight that mother pays little attention to it. Just as one example, (that will be developed further in its own section) a failure to "latch-on" in breast feeding might simply lead to immediate "bottle feeding," which seems to eliminate the problem. Therefore, depending upon the knowledge base and experience of the practitioner, obtaining all the relevant history information might require more than a bit of "digging." This is especially the case when "mild" problems are barely brought to the attention of the mother so that later, extensive developmental history data is not readily forthcoming.

However, what other variables might also play a role in defining the level of integration of a report and its usefulness for developing treatment plans? One good hunch is that a lack of application of "risk factors" for understanding a child occurs because of a *cortically-based framework* for appreciating cognition to begin with! This "best guess" warrants consideration of a few other issues. For instance, when an infant is discharged from the hospital, *medical stability* is typically assumed. However, this is not synonymous with neurodevelopmental stability and/or integrity.

Any "at risk" factors that might have initially complicated the birth history, yet were addressed in a medically appropriate way, is never a guarantee that neurodevelopmental difficulties will not occur later. The very use of the term "at risk" automatically implies that difficulties will not manifest until later. It might take several years for a neurodevelopmental deficit to manifest itself; for example, the effects of early and significant elevations in bilirubin might not be behaviorally apparent until school-age, when ADHD-like symptoms emerge [2, 3]; an infant with trouble "latching-on" or with anomalies in sucking-swallowing cycles cannot possibly exhibit "language disorder" until he/she reaches the appropriate developmental age. Furthermore, even knowing that the best trained, most qualified physician successfully treated birth-related complications says nothing about that provider's knowledge or understanding of the neuroanatomic substrates of cognitive development. There is no reason to believe any medical pediatric specialist should know about cognition. In our opinion, the rule of thumb should be, *"beware of the self-appointed expert."* An infant's discharge from the hospital does not predict anything about neurodevelopmental outcomes. This does not imply anyone did anything "wrong" or that any pediatric provider is responsible for any future developmental anomaly. However, along with hospital discharge, parents might assume their baby is "out of the woods" when in reality, that child might remain "at risk" for a less than optimal outcome for a number of years to follow! Similarly, there is a continuing, almost unshakeable "misbelief" that developmental motor and neurocognitive functions are mutually exclusive, separate and self-contained neuropsychological domains often treated as independent "compartments." Furthermore, neuroscience has developed exponentially over the span of a little over a decade! There is an ever-increasing need for translational communication; but there is no "infrastructure" of any interdisciplinary model from which to build upon for disseminating information exchange [6]. A goal of this chapter is to help close this "gap" between practitioners in various fields and even parents. Any reader, regardless of their time in practice, can likely recall at least one case when parents were "shocked" by what the neuropsychologist told them about the likely etiologies, severity, and prognostic outcome of the difficulties of their currently school-aged child. In this regard, we have an illustrative case example:

Case 1

This vignette is a case of a pre-school aged child who was diagnosed with neurofibromatosis-1 (NF-1), medically monitored at regular intervals, and seen for neuropsychological evaluation for the first time at the age of 9 years. The parents initiated the referral because they were told by school personnel there was "no reason for testing." There were numerous reasons for referral, including complaints of inattention, forgetfulness, distractibility, and a lack of progress in learning to read that was immediately evident at the age of school entry. The evaluation revealed disturbances within several dimensions of attention; objective checklists supported a behaviorally defined diagnosis of ADHD, inattentive type; language-based deficits in phonological awareness, and very slow and inaccurate performance on a subtest of continuous rapid object naming were very striking with formal scores at the 6th %ile ranking; academic achievement performances that were at the first grade level; the child met criteria for a diagnosis of Reading Disorder. However, the child's parents, both educated people of sophisticated socioeconomic status, stated they were informed by the community school system that their child was "a little slow in reading." They believed their child was struggling in all academic areas, and thought that for all practical purposes, their child was unable to read and spell. They indicated that through their independent research efforts, they learned that some children with NF-1 had learning difficulties and/or specific learning disabilities. They indicated they were told their child did not try hard enough and perhaps was "lazy." These parents were subsequently completely shattered when the neurobiology and the neuropsychology of NF-1, its general course and outcomes, was painfully discussed with them. And of course, practitioners need to come to terms with the fact that there is nothing "pretty" at all about the neuropsychological manifestations of disease processes.

It is very hard to believe that in this day and age, a case like this could ever present in this way. We completely understand that the reader might even be thinking this vignette is a fabrication! In fact, we were astonished that these parents knew about the cognitive manifestations of NF-1 only because of their own personal research efforts. There is a voluminous literature on NF-1, the associated cognitive manifestations, the subcortical anomalies that can be observed within the thalamus, basal ganglia and cerebellar regions that presumably drive the symptomatic, phenotypical presentations, and predictive data about the range of cognitive and adaptive behavioral outcomes [7–14]. However, this case literally presented in this way which is disconcerting, disturbing, and perplexing. We could not find a better case to illustrate our points if we used our "collective imagination" to simulate this presentation! But before jumping to conclusions, the facts we are illustrating are really not so bewildering. The pediatricians, neurologists, and neuroimaging experts were all doing their jobs. They executed their duties properly. However, they also unintentionally proved our point. These were top-notch service providers who were not, are not, and never conveyed the impression of being someone they were not. They defined their limits well. They knew the scope of their practices and never intended to portray any impression of expertise in cognition and/or neuropsychology. Attribution works in peculiar ways. There is no reason to indict well intentioned parents. But expertise about cognition was perhaps innocently attributed to the wrong professions.

Parents also have a nasty yet innocent habit of attributing cognitive and even neuropsychological expertise to teachers, school psychologists, learning disability instructors, and Speech/Language pathologists and Occupational Therapists who work within community school systems. Addressing these issues requires an independent, free-standing, self-contained e-book series – the issues that need coverage and explanations of the interactions between the various professions are, conveniently captured by the coined phrase, "well beyond the scope of this volume."

However, this e-book is practical, which means we are unable to ignore or shun our responsibility of discussing certain relevant issues. And the focus of this chapter, which is upon the understanding of "at risk" issues with an emphasis upon pediatric populations, unfortunately places the clinical neuropsychologist in the position of having to know about the kind of thinking that happens within community school systems. Hopefully, examining this case just a bit more will serve as an example of the need for interdisciplinary communication—by demonstrating its virtual absence!

So returning to our case example is again of clinical importance. To begin with, the professions which are found within school systems and which couldn't be of more relevance in our case example are not "experts" in neurodevelopment and/or the development of cognition. So this attribution often made by parents about community school system "professions" is a huge, unmistakable error. To put the matter bluntly, most people's "knee jerk" reaction, impetuous or perhaps even irresponsible conclusion is that the school system "dropped the ball" in our NF-1 case. Inattention, distractibility, forgetfulness; deficits in phonological processing and rapid object naming; achievement in reading at a first grade level, all identified upon formal evaluation, have nothing to do with a school-system description of a child who is "a little slow in reading." Problems within the phonological system, and deficits in rapid object naming, are the most well and consistently known "at risk" factors for reading disability which is what this chapter is all about; these "risk factors" predict deficits in the learning to read process; there was early evidence of difficulties within the learning to read process; a few years later when neuropsychological evaluation was administered, continuing deficits in reading were identified; the parents wanted "testing." For some reason, the school system saw no reason for it. Simply put, the parents were correct in their judgment; the school system could not have been more wrong! At the "risk" of being cynical, the most obvious "at risk" factor for increasing the likelihood of failing to identify deficits in cognitive development just might be *attending a school within a community school system!* Just as importantly, NF-1 is a medical condition; the cognitive manifestations of NF-1 often include deficits in attention, distractibility, and forgetfulness; the neurobiologic substrates of these symptoms include regions of the basal ganglia and the thalamus; "slowness" in learning, and in automating as manifest by diminished speed on rapid naming tasks, includes involvement of the cerebro-cerebellar circuitry system—another region of involvement in our case presentation of NF-1. Why was the ball dropped in this case? Why was time wasted before implementing an appropriate intervention?

Perhaps "the ball was not dropped?" Perhaps school system staff should be viewed much differently. Certain decisions made by the school system were based upon a flimsy understanding of learning processes. However, what if community school systems are "experts" in guiding children's learning, but only with respect to typically developing children who have no "hints" of "at risk" factors or identified cognitive deficits? What are the mechanisms which are "in place" for the translational communication that is required to keep all the practitioners involved in this case "on board" for understanding the pathology and the appropriate treatment? Perhaps the "ball" was never held? The ball was never in anyone's possession?

Solving the problems inherent in the complete mismanagement of this case clearly
illustrate the importance and relevance of this chapter! What should be commonly
known about "at risk" factors is perhaps not so commonly known! The importance
of integrating "at risk" factors with test data, practical observations of behavior,
and with known neuroanatomical substrates of behaviors is critical. This integra-
tion generates an enriched, powerful understanding of the patient which should
then lead to developing our knowledge of interventions, to understanding how these
interventions work, and in deciding upon which interventions should be applied.

And this developmental information often seems "foreign" within community
school systems as well! Absolutely no criticism intended here—it just happens; and
it happens for good reasons! But why does the cortically-based paradigm limit the
way a practitioner understands, applies, and integrates their knowledge of "at risk"
factors with neurocognitive data? The answer is deceptively simple! Just about
every "at risk" factor that is associated with neurodevelopmental outcomes is fun-
damentally grounded in brainstem, cerebellar, basal ganglia, and associated "white-
matter" tracts and functions! [15]. The generally accepted "model" *focuses upon the*
cortex. The prevailing principle assumes blatantly explicit processes are the primary drivers of behavior. Constructs such as self-control, self-awareness, and experiences of consciousness are unparalleled within this framework. When cortical
processes are accepted as "the king of the chessboard," all that really matters is the
integrity of the cortical mantle. Functions that support life, such as any and all of the
functions of the sympathetic and parasympathetic nervous systems, are clearly
indispensable. However, these functions are inexorably assigned to subcortical processes which are presumably well outside of, and separated from behaviors which
are under the influence of the "superior" human cortex. However, accepting this
"fixed assignment" theme generates an absolutely huge problem. It identifies "the
elephant within the room." It becomes impossible to consider any other pattern of
the structural organization of behavior. It is unimaginable to think about the possible role of subcortical processes in thinking; it loses phylogenetic contiguity; it
destroys the consistency of the organization of behavior along the hierarchical phylogenetic scale; and it dissociates developmental "at risk" factors from cognition;
and, it definitely makes it easy to understand a lack of any continuous relationship
between/among "at risk" factors, neurodevelopmental disorders, and the complex-
ity of human cognition. Inherent in a cortically based model is a lack of understanding of brain-behavior relationships. Finally, this places the clinician right back
where she/he started; an untenable position within which the neurodevelopment of
cognition cannot be understood.

The axiom known to many an attorney, taught early on during training, seems
important here, but only if appropriately amended. Over the course of education
and training, the aspiring lawyer is taught a simple principle: during a deposition
or trial, *never ask a question if you don't already know the answer to the question*
you are asking. The general abstraction seems to emphasize, "avoid being taken by
surprise." The astute attorney tries to "set-up" his/her case by planning a series of
questions and replies so that little, if anything, is left to chance. This principle at
least serves as a practical example of understanding the vertebrate brain as an

anticipatory control mechanism (see *The Myth of Executive Functioning* [29]). However, we want much, much more than illustrating that sample of behavior as an example of predicting anticipatory control.

This principle, if interpreted literally, does not do much for developing the proper conduct of the neuropsychologist when attempting to organize a clinical interview. However, if we adjust that principle just a little bit, we are left with a tremendously important clue; we expose a brand new way of asking efficient questions in order to obtain answers that immediately organize the clinical interview.

Neuropsychologists are compelled to ask questions about patients because they anticipate how to understand and apply the answers. There are plenty of interesting surprises that inevitably emerge; these "data points" feature vital information. So to make a question relevant, a minor but critical "twist" should always be considered within the context of what is asked about. *The purpose of any question now includes a meaningful modification which ensures the significance about what an interviewer/practitioner really wants to know.* The principle then becomes transparent!

Interviewing is a pointless exercise unless the practitioner gathers information for applying it. If the clinician does not understand the value or significance of the range of the anticipated replies, the question(s) need not be asked. The information that is revealed by the reply should be used purposefully to assist in understanding the patient. *Every question is, and should be, asked for a reason.* By simple analogy, it is accepted knowledge that an accomplished chess player should never move a chess piece unless they can verbalize the reason for making that particular move; every single move has a purpose along with anticipated outcomes. By the same token, the accomplished clinical neuropsychologist asks questions because he/she anticipates how the response will be of value. The information will always be useful, regardless of the content of the answer. The questions are always anticipatory in nature; they have a purpose. The answers provide important diagnostic clues that can assist in understanding the etiology of the given clinical presentation. Just as importantly, this information can be critical in guiding treatment. *The examiner should know the relevance and significance of all the questions and the reasons for asking them.* Neuropsychological education and training should teach the future *practitioner how to think about patients* while providing the underpinning for acquiring an ever-expanding knowledge base. To simplify the point, *do not ask questions just for the sake of asking them.* We have no concern about how a practitioner decides to waste time. However, we have every reason to be justifiably concerned about how and why any given practitioner wastes the precious commodity of the time of the patient and/or any given caregiver. At this point, we are in a position to review the usefulness of a few carefully chosen neurodevelopmental "at risk" factors. Questions about developmental "at risk" factors are always driven by purpose. The reason for asking the question is always purposeful because the answer will always generate information relevant to developmental outcomes. The questions are always related to a pattern of development that proceeds from proximal to distal brain and body regions. The questions we ask about neurodevelopmental processes are all predicated upon ontological principles including the fact that "bottom-up" developmental processes support higher-order cognitive functions.

Apgar Scores: How Are They Useful?

Apgar scores were developed by Dr. Virginia Apgar in 1952. These "scores" have been used in delivery rooms for at least 60 years. Every pediatric psychologist has heard of them, but this does not necessarily mean neuropsychologists understand them. Neuropsychologists are aware that high scores mean something good and low scores are poor, representing some sort of medical risk. To our knowledge, neuropsychologists have never been surveyed about the definition and possible significance of these scores as they understand them.

Apgar scores are sort of a health "screening test" given to infants almost immediately after birth. These scores, organized along a 10-point scale, are a rough index of post-birth health. These scores are derived from five clinical signs, specifically, heart rate, respiratory effort, reflex irritability, muscle tone, and color. These areas are intended to represent the "vital signs" of infancy. The initial observations of the circulatory and pulmonary systems generate data about the fundamentals that support life; rough observations of the motor system are to provide an index of motor integrity; a superficial observation of color can provide a clue about possible jaundice. Every "sign" is assigned a value ranging from 0 to 2; any total score within the range of 7–10 falls within the normal range. These Apgar ratings are made at 1 and 5 minutes after birth. When an infant requires supportive medical services, these ratings might be repeated again, at 10 and 20 minutes.

The value of Apgar scores as a possible predictor of later-onset disabilities has been debated. Scores between 8 and 10 are interpreted as signs of good infant health. The majority of infants with scores of 7 do perfectly fine. Overall, Apgar scores tell us very little when considered in isolation; the *reason* for the low score is the more important factor, and this is usually observed by additional symptoms. Scores in the intermediate range of 4–6 after 5 minutes, coupled with neonatal symptoms, are often associated with an increased risk of later-onset neurodevelopmental disorders; scores between 0 and 3, along with the subsequent observance of neonatal encephalopathy, are much more often associated with developmental disorders [16].

A Selective Review of Basic Developmental "At Risk" Factors

Much of this information was reviewed in *ADHD as a Model of Brain-Behavior Relationships* [28] and *The Myth of Executive Functioning* [29]. However, since we reviewed the how and why of asking "anticipatory questions" in the aforementioned text, this selective review of certain concepts provides a useful opportunity for completing our theme. Since we develop from proximal to distal regions, and since phylogenetically older brain regions develop before newer neocortical areas, it makes sense that the level of development of the cerebellum would be an important driver of early behavior [17]. One of the oldest regions of the cerebellum, the vestibular cerebellum, is considered mature at 40 weeks gestation. While this implicates the importance of the cerebellum in overall neurodevelopmental processes, other data speak directly to this point. Limperopoulos and colleagues [18] found that full-term infants with cerebellar injury at the time of delivery exhibited a broad spectrum of neurodevelopmental disabilities, including motor anomalies. Early motor development predicts later development, including performance on complex cognitive tasks of working memory and related executive functions [19]. Therefore, both cerebellar and motor anomalies should be considered "at risk" factors for the development of later cognitive anomalies.

There are many other very commonly known "at risk" factors that can affect pre- and post-natal development. For example, the negative effects of smoking and/or consuming alcohol/illicit substances during pregnancy are very well known and include low birth weight and/or fetal alcohol syndrome. Other gestational circumstances include poor nutrition, level of pre-natal care, general maternal health, and the psychosocial well-being of the mother. Some "at risk" factors have been studied more comprehensively than others. However, premature delivery has arguably been investigated more than any other factor.

Premature Birth

Length of pregnancy as it pertains to fetal and later neurodevelopment is not nearly as controversial as it was in the past. For example, a 37–38 weeks gestation is typically considered sufficient for medical stability; however, this is not necessarily the case from a neuropsychological point of view. It has been documented through specialized neuro-imaging technologies that a 37 weeks gestation can be associated with the development of micro-structural changes within the brain, regardless of the neonate's level of medical stability [20]. At 37–38 weeks the vestibular cerebellum is not mature, birth automatically slows down brain maturation processes, so it becomes important to apply this information for understanding pediatric presentations [21]. A gestational term of 37–38 weeks already increases the likelihood of cognitive disorder at school age, and even a poorer longer-term neurocognitive outcome [21].

Birth prior to 37 weeks' gestation is considered preterm, or premature, and birth at 32 weeks gestation or less is termed very premature. The American College of Obstetricians and Gynecologists advises against non-medically indicated birth prior to 39 weeks' gestation [22]. A voluminous literature describes and characterizes the risk factors associated with preterm birth. For example, low birth weight, jaundice, feeding problems, and peri-ventricular leukomalacia (PVL) are more common in preterm infants [1, 23]. Preterm birth also increases the risk of complications during delivery, which then further increases the likelihood for atypical neurodevelopment [24]. As a general rule that nearly always holds true, preterm and/or very preterm birth are associated with multiple "at risk" factors that often impact upon cognitive development and longer-term outcomes. Within our outline for gathering information, we move from asking questions about "at risk" factors towards obtaining objective documentation from other sources. Since the length of time that passed over the years can easily distort anyone's recollection, reviewing objective records can reveal more substantive information. By definition, prematurity almost never occurs in isolation. Reports from providers that participated in early interventions are often useful.

Twin gestation is almost always associated with preterm birth [25] and is frequently associated with additional factors such as breach presentation. Achievement of 38 weeks' gestation in twin pregnancies is considered medically adequate, but this again does not necessarily imply later cognitive integrity. Breach presentation increases the likelihood of hip dysplasia. In turn, this can compromise movement, which then can compromise cognitive integrity. Fetal position is also important during the course of gestation as it arguably supports the foundation for balance for the developing vestibular system [25]. It also remains unclear as to whether or not this might be associated with an increased likelihood of anxiety disorders. However, anomalous development of the vestibular system can impact upon the achievement of the typical developmental motor milestones of sitting independently, crawling, walking, and language acquisition [26]. Since cognitive control is an "extension" of motor control, anomalous motor development often corresponds with the integrity of metacognitive functions, regardless of the etiology of compromised movement [3, 17, 19, 27].

Feeding, Language, and Reward

There is a very close relationship between early motor development and the integrity of "executive functions." The "chain of events" that link early motor abilities with the development of thinking have been summarized in *The Myth of Executive Functioning* [29] of this series [29]. This theoretical linkage has also been reviewed by Koziol and Lutz [17] as well as by Koziol, Budding, and Chidekel [27]. Longitudinal investigations with quantifiable test score relationships served as the direct foundational evidence which supported further theoretical conclusions. At this stage, in the practical academic and clinical settings, the relationship between motor control and cognitive control should be considered unequivocal, undeniable, generally accepted knowledge. These relationships were initially hypothesized; later systematic investigations generated a voluminous supportive literature; finally, the data were combined, in aggregate, as unmistakable conclusions emerged [19, 30–35]. *Knowing about early and ongoing motor development not only informs us, but allows us to predict the integrity of executive functions or "cognitive control."*

Nevertheless, despite the weight of the evidence, these concepts seem foreign with respect to practical applications. We have already explained why this "disconnect" exists between the science of the matter and actual practice, but it is worth noting again, since repetition leads to "remembering"; first, the tendency to place "related" functions within artificially constructed, arbitrary domains is unshakable; second, supposedly "higher-order" functions are considered a manifestation of neocortical processes, superior to "rudimentary" subcortical controls.

Motor ability is evident early on during the course of the pregnancy; the "moving and kicking" experienced by the mother is literally a manifestation of reflex activity [26]. Movement is immediately evident at birth. The symptom of hypotonia is often identified very early, and children with low muscle tone demonstrate poorer cognitive outcomes as adults. Yet one of the earliest indices that *predict* neuromotor integrity and the later development of cognitive control is frequently overlooked. An infant's ability to suck predicts cognitive developmental outcomes [36]. Difficulties in "latching on," weak sucking strength, disturbances in sucking and swallowing cycles, and in aggregate, a lack of coordination within these processes are the harbinger of poor neurodevelopmental outcomes.

Upon interview with a parent, difficulties in these areas are frequently denied right from the start. Considerable questioning in this area, with highly specific probing, is often necessary for useful information to emerge. As the aforementioned text reviewed, feeding problems might be denied because the mother might have claimed she was "nervous," and that immediately switching to "bottle feeding" solved the problem. Another answer that might emerge is that intubation was required for a brief post-natal period, and when the "tube" was removed, there were absolutely no identifiable problems in latching on, sucking, or swallowing. These recollections might be exactly right. However, any obstruction within the mouth can very easily disrupt, or temporarily disturb, the natural progression of the development of the oromotor musculature [37]. This is particularly notable in cases of premature birth; in fact, according to Amaizu and colleagues [38], gestational age by itself is a *direct predictor* of nutritive sucking abilities.

Failure to latch-on during feeding has been specifically associated with a significantly increased likelihood of developmental speech/language disturbances [36]. In fact, this is perhaps one of the most reliable predictors that can be asserted with respect to longer-term developmental speech/language problems. Because these factors can be pertinent signs that predict the need for later intervention, they simply cannot be overlooked. But regardless of the persuasiveness of the evidence, people do not pay much attention to it. Assuming the cortex is disproportionately so important neglects the fact that descending cortical input, intact brainstem mechanisms, and reciprocal connections with the cerebellum support early feeding, while these same brain regions overlap with the cortical, subcortical, and brainstem regions recruited for speech and language production [4, 39, 40]. This is but one dramatic illustration of how a cortico-centric bias can limit our understanding of brain-behavior relationships as well as an opportunity to provide an early intervention.

The brain is an anticipatory control mechanism that functions on the basis of expectation or prediction. This also has relevance for the reward system, as was indicated in the *The Myth of Executive Functioning* [29]. Systematic investigations concerning feeding behavior and the development of reward circuitry systems has not been conducted; however, the purpose of the suck reflex is to anticipate food and nurturance (i.e., reward) [41]. Based upon these basic principles, one might also expect that difficulties with reflexive latching-on, sucking, and swallowing cycles might have a negative impact upon the development of reward systems as well. This is a matter that requires systematic investigation. We have all seen patients who have difficulties initiating interactions with others and interacting with examiners, despite being completely cooperative. These patients give the impression of lacking initiative and motivation, and many appear to have a limited range of interests. It is certainly plausible that this relates to early feeding patterns and their potential relation to the development of reward systems. Therefore, even a seemingly simple behavior, like a reflex, can have a profound impact upon brain development with respect to a wide variety of longer-term cognitive and behavioral outcomes. This might even extend to include a-motivational syndromes and the development of negative and positive reward preferences [41]. Therefore, by dismantling the cortico-centric perspective, by including and studying brainstem, cerebellar, and basal contributions to development and cognition, we open new doors for generating hypotheses about important aspects of behavioral adaptation that should lead to systematic investigations to enhance our knowledge base; this should invariably lead to a better understanding of development and new treatment approaches.

Hyperbilirubinemia

Jaundice is another factor which is frequently minimized, even though it occurs in approximately 60 % of births [42]. According to a review by Koziol and colleagues [3] it is generally accepted that moderate elevations in bilirubin are associated with a general "at risk" factor for cognitive, perceptual, motor, and auditory disorders. Furthermore, elevations in bilirubin (defined as moderate, at the 95th %ile), place neonates "at risk" for a subsequent diagnosis of attention deficit hyperactivity disorder, autism spectrum disorders, central auditory processing disorders, and/or generalized academic learning difficulties [43–45]. In aggregate, these groups of symptoms and disorders are frequently categorized under the generalized term of BINDS, or Bilirubin Induced Neurologic Dysfunction [3]. Alternatively, these conditions are classified as partial kernicterus syndromes.

Several specific "subcortical" regions of the brain are *spontaneously active* before birth, as well as during and after the birth process and throughout adulthood. As previously reviewed, these regions include the basal ganglia, but more specifically, the Globus Pallidus interna, or GPi; the GPi plays a very special role. For example, the cerebral cortex needs to be activated in order for it to perform its highly specialized activities. Obviously, all perceptions, and/or actions, should not and cannot be activated simultaneously in order for purposive, goal-directed, highly selective behaviors to be executed. The GPi, through its constant firing upon the thalamus, prevents the thalamus from activating the cortex, therefore preventing behavioral release. In order for an appropriate behavior to be selected, the GPi "stops" inhibiting the appropriate thalamic nuclei, enabling that particular focused behavior to be executed, or released. The dentate nucleus of the cerebellum also projects to the thalamus; the cerebellum adjusts behaviors along a hierarchically organized "metric." All sensory experiences, and all actions, must be adjusted so that within any situation, the sensory function is not too strong, nor is it too weak; for instance, imagine the experiences of touch sensation; the experience of emotion; the sensation of sounds and the intensity of lighting conditions; ideally, all of these "perceptions" are experienced in a way that is "just right,"…, not too strong; not too weak. When playing a piano, or using a computer keyboard, the "keys" should be touched with just the right amount of force. So the dentate nucleus of the cerebellum is always sending neural signals through the thalamus and then on to the cortex to adjust the appropriate rate, rhythm, and force of a behavior. The hippocampus must also be spontaneously active, and appropriately "inhibited," to encode or regulate the proper sensory experiences to be appropriately registered within the cortex so that later, the experience can be recalled with sufficient detail, integration, and clarity. The point here concerns the "facts" that these spontaneously active brain regions perform their respective roles properly— this always requires the appropriate "balance" between neural activation and neural inhibition [42, 46–51] Granted, these examples are rudimentary, but this is exactly the simplicity that is intended to understand these possibly "novel" patterns.

In cases of jaundice, these brain regions, which are all *spontaneously active within their default mode (when the brain is presumably at rest)* receive less "nutrient;" moderately high levels of bilirubin (defined as levels which reach the 95th %ile) *are replacing oxygen content within the bloodstream* [2, 3]. Even these over-simplified examples provided a sufficient framework for understanding how cell death, as the result of hyperbilirubinemia generating necrotic brain tissue, significantly compromises those groups of nuclei that demand the most oxygen/nutrient in order to perform their critical inhibitory functions. Therefore, during a clinical interview, there are numerous reasons for asking about jaundice, levels of bilirubin concentration, the duration of jaundice, and the type, and length of interventions that were required. Answers to these questions place the case presentation within clinical context. And this means there is every reason for integrating this information into a neuropsychology report.

Prenatal Reflexes: Why Are They Important?

All sensorimotor activity is purposeful [30, 52, 53]; there is nothing random about it. Simple reflexes, such as the suck reflex, are significant because they predict an outcome. Before birth, movement within the womb is not random—these are infant reflexes that at the very minimum serve the purpose of "exercise." [54]. It is no accident that babies who are "inactive" before birth often exhibit the symptom of hypotonia. Low muscle tone can occur for a variety reasons, but most of these reasons are brain-related and later during the course of development are associated with poor control over the motor system. Furthermore, poor control over the motor system is symptomatic of poor cognitive control. Children with idiopathic hypotonia have poorer cognitive outcomes as compared to their typically developing peers [55]. Deficits in motor coordination, language, and general learning difficulties are common problems that persist within this group.

The Progression from Sitting to Crawling to Walking: Why Is This Important?

Attention, Balance and Coordination: The A.B.C.'s of Learning Success [26] is arguably the most comprehensive review of the primitive and transitional reflexes observed across the lifespan. Although we never intended an extensive review of these reflexes, some of these reflexes play an important role and are observed in typically developing children as they progress through the pattern of the "traditional" developmental milestones; similarly, the disinhibition of reflexes that once served a purpose in infancy and/or early childhood are often observed in school-aged children diagnosed with pathologies such as ADHD [15]. In this section, we review two important "transitional" reflexes because of their developmental importance and observed frequency.

We were born to move! Perhaps the most obvious feature of infant behavior is movement. Any attentive observer will immediately notice that an infant not only moves with notable frequency, but also almost never moves one limb at a time, individually, in isolation. Instead, we observe that the upper limbs move with the lower limbs, and the head moves with the limbs, in combinations. This is not accidental. In a newborn infant, the musculature of the head, the upper limbs, and the lower limbs are coupled together in various reflexive patterns [56]. The "job" of the developing child is to acquire control over the motor system. One critical step in developing motor control is separating these innately coupled movements. In this regard, sitting independently, crawling, and walking are important underpinnings of this developmental control process. Two important reflexes often observed during this process are the asymmetric tonic neck reflex (ATNR) and the symmetric tonic neck reflex (STNR).

The ATNR is evident before birth in response to rotation, emerging somewhere around 18–20 weeks of gestation [57]. This development coincides with the time mothers often begin to notice a baby's movements. Rotation of the infant's head toward one side is followed by extension of the arm and leg on the same side, and a retraction of the opposite arm [57]. This reflex grows stronger throughout the course of the pregnancy [57], and it serves different purposes at different times. The ATNR helps the fetus to move around within the womb—to turn, to exercise muscles, and to adjust its position in response to the mother's movements. The fetus specifically adapts to the mother's changes in posture [58]. It is assumed that this occurs so that the fetus can make itself comfortable, in order to exercise fetal musculature, and even to explore its tiny world [58]. The ATNR also helps to develop independent movements on each side of the body [57]. It has been proposed that, during the course of delivery, it is the ATNR that helps the infant adjust its position in order to assist in the birthing process [57]. After this reflex has served its purpose, it is suppressed or inhibited [57]. It re-emerges at different times. It is no accident that infants born "floppy," with hypotonia or low muscle tone, are often described as not being very active during the course of the pregnancy; they have not had the benefit of this exercise.

The ATNR, after delivery, is also expressed when the baby lies on its stomach [59]. More specifically, this reflex is released in order to ensure that the infant's head turns to one side to free the airway for breathing [59]. Early inhibition of this reflex is believed to be an underpinning of sudden infant death syndrome, or SIDS. These examples also illustrate that movement always serves a purpose.

As a brief summary, the ATNR ensures that when the head is turned, not only do the arms stretch out on the same side, but the eyes also move in the same direction as the head and arm [59]. In this way, the ATNR may impact the infant's visual domain as the infant focuses upon near points (e.g., when the head is in the middle and the hands are in front of the face), which hypothetically has the potential to influence the development of the ventral and dorsal attention networks. As the head turns and the eyes follow the direction of the extending arm and hand, the development of the ventral attention network is, hypothetically, influenced. The attentive reader who has read the previously mentioned volumes will recall that the ventral attention network focuses upon allocentric space (i.e., distance), while the dorsal attention network focuses upon egocentric space (i.e., nearby). Allocentric space includes objects outside of an individual's immediate reach or grasp, while egocentric space includes objects and items within an individual's immediate reach or grasp. Therefore, as a very general principle, the ATNR can be understood as having an influence on the early development of attention-related processes and behavioral control; however, with inhibitory failures, the ATNR can remain active [57]. When this occurs, the arm stretches out when the head is turned to the side. This makes it particularly difficult to bring the hand to the nose, or to the midline, which can then influence development of the dorsal attention network. The ATNR is typically fully inhibited at approximately 6 months after birth [26].

Poor integration of reflex control is often observed in neurodevelopmental disorders of disinhibition, such as ADHD [15, 23, 60–63]. In fact, disinhibition is observed in a variety of disorders, and this can include disinhibition of the ATNR. Therefore, we would expect a hyperactive ventral attention network resulting in increased focus upon items and events in allocentric space, but a difficulty in achieving balance with the dorsal attention network [64]. Therefore, the child becomes overly focused upon what is within allocentric space, looking around instead of what is in front of him/her, resulting in a possible contributor to off-task behavior. In other words, this represents a type of distractibility. It becomes extremely difficult for the child to develop fine motor control when this occurs, which can result in the expression of poor executive direction and control over fine motor movement. As the head turns, the tendency is to extend the arm. This can affect pencil grip as the pencil might be controlled with whole-arm movements, instead of with the coordination of the wrists and finger tips. Ordinarily, the DAN informs frontal systems about the parameters for *how* to perform the pencil movements. This requires balanced interactions between the VAN and DAN. A lack of suppression of the ATNR might prove to represent a useful, observable index of an overactive VAN. These remain clinical hypotheses derived from expectations about brain network interactions that warrant systematic investigations in order to better understand neurodevelopment.

The STNR appears strongly at about 8 months of age [26]. It is initially observed when the infant starts to push itself up off the ground from a prone position [26]. This is in preparation for creeping and crawling on the hands and knees. When the infant lifts or extends its head up, the movement is accompanied by an extension of the upper limbs, and a flexion of the lower limbs [26]. When the head looks down in a flexion position, the limbs of the upper body also flex, and the lower limbs extend [26]. The STNR not only supports the evolving ability of crawling, which is considered critical to the exploratory behavior which theoretically supports the development of ventral and dorsal attention networks.

These general purposes of the STNR can be further sub-divided. First, infants make purposive movements that reflect a coupling of the upper and lower limbs. This was observed in the description of the ATNR, and it is similarly evident in the STNR, but in a different way. One function of the STNR is to provide the exercise necessary to completely decouple head movement from upper and lower limb movements, so that eventually all limbs can function and move independently [56]. Therefore, crawling represents a huge step in the child's ability to acquire control over the motor system. Once again, the critical development of "action control" is readily observed. This type of separation is similarly necessary for the subsequent development of fine motor control, again reflecting the proximal to distal developmental relationship. This further illustrates the "job" of the typically developing child as the process of acquiring increasing control over the motor system.

Hypothetically, one would expect a strong relationship between the STNR and the development of the dorsal and ventral attention networks [65]. To reiterate, the ventral attention network focuses upon objects in allocentric space, while the dorsal attention network focuses upon egocentric space. A focus on allocentric space is related to the development of the reward system. The ventral attention network, sometimes referred to as the "what" pathway, supports object identification—the reason for object identification is to associate objects with appropriate reward value [66] as already described in the the previously mentioned volumes. In other words, we recognize objects because of their worth, because we know what they can be used for in fulfilling a need, or for the purpose of protection. We learn to approach those objects that are of immediate positive reward value, and we learn to avoid those objects that generate fear or anxiety. This is a basal ganglia governed instrumental learning process; as reviewed in volume II, the basal ganglia learn what to do and what not to do, a process which is critical for adaptation/survival. The VAN provides reward information and therefore, the ventral attention network is strongly related to our development of interests, and our ability to sustain attention to those interests. A child's initial ability to move, and in this case crawl, is the underpinning of approach-avoidance behavior acquired through VAN-motor system interactions.

The dorsal attention network focuses upon egocentric space, and has been referred to as the "where" pathway. The dorsal attention network, with its neuroanatomical localization within the frontal eye fields and the parietal lobes, specify the "parameters of action". This means that the DAN provides information to the frontal lobes about "how" to interact with, or use those objects in order for them to be useful to us. Therefore, interactions between the VAN and the DAN represent the neuro-anatomic substrate for "action control." Crawling provides an early under-pinning of action control as the VAN and DAN interact for the child's exploratory behavior. These interactions can be inferred by taking a closer look at crawling behavior.

For example, in crawling, when the head extends looking away or upward, the child's focus is on allocentric space, hypothetically activating the ventral attention network (specifically the temporal lobes and associated regions as described in previous volumes of this series). When the head and neck flex downward during crawling, or when the infant looks down, the focus shifts to egocentric space, pre-sumably activating the dorsal attention network. Therefore, the STNR, observed in crawling, not only serves the purpose of separating head from limb movements, but it also supports dynamic VAN-DAN interactions which eventually generates early instrumental learning. As a child explores his or her environment, finding objects of interest, and then focusing immediate attention upon these objects to play with them, approach-avoidance behaviors are acquired and action control is developed. This represents early "executive functioning," or what we prefer to call cognitive or action control.

Additionally, inherent in the exercise of decoupling the head from upper and lower limb movements is the critical idea of motor programming. Crawling requires the proper sequencing and ordering of movements. In order to crawl, the proper sequence must be established and performed in the same way, every time, in proper order. This eventually leads to automatic crawling. This might be con-sidered the forerunner of automaticity. The typically developing child quickly learns to crawl, while looking at something else, evaluating or remembering its significance or reward value as the child moves toward an object of interest. In this way, crawling, or automating a proper motor sequence or motor program, further establishes an aspect of the platform for the development of executive functioning, cognitive control, or thinking. In other words, this lays the founda-tion for the proper ordering of ideas when thinking. In this way, thinking repre-sents action control, or control over the motor system. In this regard, the purpose of all thinking is the control of action.

Thoughts represent sequences of movement that will later be performed as we interact with any given set of circumstances, as we constantly interact within a dynamically changing environment. We are always moving through space in some way, shape, or form, and we always continually interact with objects in our world. Much of what we do on a daily basis, perhaps 95 % of our activities, are based upon automatic behavior [67], or things that we do on a regular basis. Problem-solving, and the thinking it requires, is nothing more than imagining and ordering ideas that are later translated into necessary movements. The behavior becomes automatic the more often the activities are repeated, or performed. In this way, crawling and its relationship to the development of cognitive control as we have defined and described it, is fundamental to perception-action coupling. This "coupling" is the "work" within the concept of "working memory."

Additional Case Presentations

This chapter provided a brief review of certain important developmental concepts. The purpose of this presentation was to emphasize how developmental history data might be used to assist in identifying symptoms and to use these data for generating an integrated understanding a person. The following case vignettes provide practical examples:

Case 2: An Erroneous and Misleading History

This is the case of a 15 year-old female. She presents with poor motivation, a lack of interest, and poor academic functioning. The results of the original neuropsychological assessment were considered inconclusive. She was seen for a second opinion approximately 1 year later because her difficulties persisted.

The initial neuropsychological assessment described an essentially unremarkable history. The report indicated there were absolutely no neurodevelopmental difficulties. The report also stated the medical history was within normal limits and non-contributory. In fact, the entire history was termed "unremarkable." The patient was administered a variety of neuropsychological tests. The results of that evaluation were considered inconclusive with respect to a differential diagnosis. In a subsequent chapter, it will be demonstrated how those data were anything but inconclusive, and how combining this data with neuropsychological history would in fact identify and explain numerous symptoms, as well as lead to appropriate treatment recommendations; however, for now, the discussion is restricted to the accuracy of the historic data.

A completely different history was obtained when the patient presented for a second opinion. There were numerous inaccuracies from the first evaluation. It is true that the pregnancy was considered "normal," but it was, in fact, not a typical pregnancy. For example, at 24–25 weeks' gestation, the patient's mother experienced pre-term labor, and steroid medications were prescribed for approximately 1 week to prevent early delivery. It remains debatable as to whether or not steroid administration during labor may reduce the rate of brain development [68]; therefore, prescription of steroid medication in this case may be considered a potential risk factor for increasing the likelihood of neurodevelopmental disorder.

The previous evaluation stated that early developmental motor milestones were accomplished within normal limits, on time, and without any neurodevelopmental delay. Further interview revealed that this was, in fact, untrue. The patient actually never crawled. In addition, while the initial evaluation stated that, "developmental history does not appear significant," this statement was also far from the truth. The patient's mother reported the patient demonstrated difficulties with inattention and maintaining age-appropriate academic motivation beginning in the third to fourth grade. This information was obtained directly from parental report during the course of standard history-taking. We have no explanation as to how or why this critical information was not "known" at the time of the prior, first assessment.

The medical history was anything but insignificant. The patient possibly experienced a traumatic brain injury in the form of a concussion approximately 7 months before the first neuropsychological assessment was completed. She was involved in a physical education accident at school in which she fell and hit her head. There was no loss of consciousness, but she was taken to the hospital. The medical records, obtained during the course of the subsequent evaluation for the "second opinion," indicated the patient experienced several symptoms of concussion and recommended she be monitored for possible symptomatic progression. These symptoms included a sense of shock and "disorientation." The symptoms that were observed quickly remitted. Approximately 5 months later, the patient was involved in a second accident in which another concussion was suspected. Immediately after this second concussion, the patient was taken to hospital, and a CT scan was administered. The results of that scan were inconsistent with what would be observed in an individual with a concussion.

However, the CT scan identified a prominent cavum velum interpositum. This lesion was described as rather large—nearly 3 cm in width—and was not associated with hydrocephalus. It was described as a midline cyst, which is a very rare type of brain anomaly that is usually found incidentally, just as it was in this particular case. This type of lesion is almost always medically stable; however, it is important to keep in mind that medical stability does not necessarily rule out cognitive symptomatology, nor does it predict cognitive outcome. In short, medical stability does not equate to efficiency of adaptive cognition. This finding represents a very subtle issue that can easily be overlooked during the course of reviewing a patient's history.

Although the actual neuropsychological data are not being reviewed within this vignette, the original results were far from inconclusive. In addition, results obtained during the second opinion evaluation were not within normal limits, and identified numerous cognitive deficiencies that were clinically significant. Perhaps the most significant point to be made in regard to reviewing the history is that the developmental and subsequent medical history that were obtained were highly significant, and certainly consistent with certain aspects of the patient's presentation. For example, the patient presented with a lack of motivation and interest, apathy, and even was diagnosed with depression; however, it remains extremely curious that the CT scan identified significant information, specifically a midline cyst that could easily cause the patient's presenting symptom picture. Similarly, the fact that this individual's difficulties were of early onset was completely overlooked in the initial evaluation, to the extent that the diagnosis was completely misleading. The patient's history is actually correct in pointing towards attention-related deficits, while the identified midline lesion could easily be a contributor to the chronic symptom picture.

Case 3

This case vignette concerns an 11 year-old female. Her developmental history is quite significant. First, she had a weak suck reflex as an infant. She was late in meeting all developmental motor milestones. For example, she sat independently at approximately 9 months. She was diagnosed with the symptom of hypotonia (i.e., low muscle tone), and she did not crawl, but instead, she scooted. The patient has never been able to ride a two-wheeled bicycle, and at present she can only ride a three-wheeler. She has been described as chronically clumsy, unable to hop on one foot, unable to skip, and tending to trip while walking. She also has extremely poor handwriting. The patient continues to experience articulation difficulties, and she is a literal thinker, inclined to interpret language concretely, without elaboration or age-appropriate abstraction. It is also potentially notable that she was the product of an artificially inseminated pregnancy.

The developmental data is obviously significant. It remains debatable as to whether or not artificial insemination increases the likelihood of neurodevelopmental disorders, but can at least be considered a potential risk factor. It is notable that she had difficulties with latching-on and feeding cycles, because this child went on to develop language difficulties. Not only has she had persistent articulation deficits, but she was unable to speak single sounds until she was 12 months old. She was slow to learn the alphabet, colors, and counting.

During the course of the evaluation, she demonstrated obvious difficulties in sustaining attention to various testing tasks. She displayed poor posture, and she was frequently observed leaning on the arms of her chair or on the table when she was asked or required to maintain an upright seated position. Language fluency difficulties were also observed. Once again, she had difficulties when asked to stand or hop on one foot at a time. She also had poor coordination when she was asked to simply hop with both feet. She had difficulties walking backwards. The patient continues to display difficulties with procedural learning and memory. For example, she has not yet acquired automated personal hygiene and dressing behavior. Many of these observations might immediately be predicted on the basis of the historic information that was obtained.

Discussion

CASE II was "easy" to interpret. The case obviously demonstrated "poor" vs. "better" history taking. Perhaps nearly everyone reading this volume has been asked to provide a second opinion on a clinical case. Readers should ask themselves how many times they have noted such inaccuracy in obtaining historic information, and how unnecessary a second opinion would be if adequate historical information was taken and correctly interpreted during the initial evaluation. The fact that this case occurred as it was reported demonstrates the range of variability in the competence levels of practitioners in clinical neuropsychology. Unfortunately, the profession has no accepted way to monitor this type of variability or to prevent it.

CASE III was perhaps of greater clinical interest. Minimal interpretation was offered, but the purpose in presenting it was quite simple; hopefully, the point was made that knowledge and its appropriate application are powerful clinical tools. We presented an exercise for the reader to interpret practical clinical information. There is much to be gained from learning how to solve clinical problems of ambiguity.

References

1. Riva, D., Bulgheroni, S., Usilla, A., Treccani, C., Saletti, V., Esposito, S., & Vago, C. (2000). Brain alterations in preterm infants: Long-term cognitive and neuropsychological outcomes. In: D. Riva & C. Njiokiktjien (Eds.), *Brain lesion localization and developmental functions* (pp. 55–64). Montrouge, France: John Libbey Eurotext.
2. Koziol, L. F., Budding, D. E., & Chidekel, D. (2013). Hyperbilirubinemia: Subcortical mechanisms of cognitive and behavioral dysfunction. *Pediatric Neurology, 48*, 3–13.
3. Koziol, L. F., & Barker, L. A. (2013). Hypotonia, jaundice, and Chiari malformations: Relationships to executive functions. *Applied Neuropsychology Child, 2*(2), 141–149.
4. Koziol, L. F., Barker, L. A., & Jansons, L. (2016). Conceptualizing developmental language disorders: A theoretical framework including the role of the cerebellum in language-related functioning. In P. Marien & M. Manto (Eds.), *The linguistic cerebellum*. San Diego, CA: Academic Press.
5. Voeller, K. K. (2004). Attention-deficit hyperactivity disorder (ADHD). *Journal of Child Neurology, 19*(10), 798–814.
6. Hastings, J., Frishkoff, G. A., Smith, B., Jensen, M., Poldrack, R. A., Lomax, J., … Martone, M. E. (2014). Interdisciplinary perspectives on the development, integration, and application of cognitive ontologies. *Frontiers in Neuroinformatics, 8*, 62.
7. Klein-Tasman, B. P., Janke, K. M., Luo, W., Casnar, C. L., Hunter, S. J., Tonsgard, J., … Kais, L. A. (2014). Cognitive and psychosocial phenotype of young children with neurofibromatosis-1. *Journal of the International Neuropsychological Society, 20*(1), 88–98.
8. Costa, R. M., & Silva, A. J. (2002). Molecular and cellular mechanisms underlying the cognitive deficits associated with neurofibromatosis-1. *Journal of Child Neurology, 17*(8), 622–626.
9. Cutting, L. E., Clements, A. M., Lightman, A. D., Yerby-Hammack, P. D., & Denckla, M. B. (2004). Cognitive profile of neurofibromatosis type 1: Rethinking nonverbal learning disabilities. *Learning Disabilities Research and Practice, 19*(3), 155–165.
10. Hyman, S. L., Shores, A., & North, K. N. (2005). The nature and frequency of cognitive deficits in children with neurofibromatosis type 1. *Neurology, 65*(7), 1037–1044.
11. Hyman, S. L., Shores, A., & North, K. N. (2006). Learning disabilities in children with neurofibromatosis type 1: Subtypes, cognitive profile, and attention-deficit-hyperactivity disorder. *Developmental Medicine and Child Neurology, 48*(12), 973–977.
12. Mazzocco, M. M., Turner, J. E., Denckla, M. B., Hoffman, R. O., Scanlon, D., & Vellutino, F. (1995). Language and reading deficits associated with neurofibromatosis type 1. *Developmental Neuropsychology, 11*, 503–522.
13. Soucy, E. A., Gao, F., Gutmann, D. H., & Dunn, C. M. (2012). Developmental delays in children with neurofibromatosis type 1. *Journal of Child Neurology, 27*(5), 641–644.
14. Barton, B., & North, K. (2004). Social skills of children with neurofibromatosis type 1. *Developmental Medicine and Child Neurology, 46*, 553–563.
15. Konicarova, J., & Bob, P. (2013). Principle of dissolution and primitive reflexes in ADHD. *Activas Nervosa Superior, 55*(1–2), 74–78.

16. Moster, D., Lie, R., & Markestad, T. (2002). Joint association of Apgar scores and early neo-natal symptoms with minor disabilities at school age. *Archives of Disease in Childhood. Fetal and Neonatal Edition, 86*(1), F16–F21. Retrieved from http://doi.org/10.1136/fn.86.1.F16
17. Koziol, L. F., & Lutz, J. T. (2013). From movement to thought: The development of executive function. *Applied Neuropsychology Child, 2*(2), 104–115.
18. Limperopoulos, C., Robertson, R. L., Sullivan, N. R., Bassan, H., & du Plessis, A. J. (2009). Cerebellar injury in term infants: Clinical characteristics, magnetic resonance imaging find-ings, and outcome. *Pediatric Neurology, 41*(1), 1–8. doi:10.1016/j.pediatrneurol.2009.02.007.
19. Piek, J. P., Dawson, L., Smith, L. M., & Gasson, N. (2008). The role of early fine and gross motor development on later motor and cognitive ability. *Human Movement Science, 27*(5), 668–681.
20. Broekman, B.F., Wang, C., Li, Y., Rifkin-Graboi, A., Saw, S.M., Chong, Y., … Qiu A. (2014). Gestational age and neonatal brain microstructure in term born infants: A birth cohort study. *PLoS One, 9*(12), e115229.
21. Kurjak, A., Antsaklis, P., & Stanojevic, M. (2015). Fetal neurology: Past, present and future. *Donald School Journal of Ultrasound in Obstetrics and Gynecology, 9*(1), 6–29.
22. Nonmedically indicated early-term deliveries. Committee Opinion No. 561. American College of Obstetricians and Gynecologists. (2013). *Obstetrics & Gynecology, 121*, 911–915.
23. Kugelman, A., & Colin, A. A. (2013). Late preterm infants: Near term but still in a critical development time period. *Pediatrics, 132*(4), 741–751.
24. Behrman, R. E., Butler, A. S. (Eds.); Institute of Medicine (US) Committee on Understanding Premature Birth and Assuring Healthy Outcomes. (2007). *Preterm birth: Causes, conse-quences, and prevention.* Washington, DC: National Academies Press (US).
25. Montgomery, K. S., Cubera, S., Belcher, C., Patrick, D., Funderburk, H., Melton, C., & Fastenau, M. (2005). Childbirth education for multiple pregnancy: Part 1: Prenatal Considerations. *The Journal of Perinatal Education, 14*(2), 26–35. doi:10.1624/105812405X44709
26. Blythe, S. (2009). *Attention, balance, and coordination: The A.B.C. of learning success.* Chichester, England: Wiley-Blackwell.
27. Koziol, L. F., Budding, D. E., & Chidekel, D. (2012). From movement to thought: Executive function, embodied cognition, and the cerebellum. *Cerebellum, 11*(2), 505–525.
28. ADHD as a Model of Brain -Behavior Relationships.
29. Koziol, L. F. (2014). *The myth of executive functioning: Missing elements in conceptualiza-tion, evaluation, and assessment.* New York, NY: Springer.
30. Von Hofsten, C. (2007). Action in development. *Developmental Science, 10*(1), 54–60.
31. Westendorp, M., Hartman, E., Houwen, S., Smith, J., & Visscher, C. (2011). The relationship between gross motor skills and academic achievement in children with learning disabilities. *Research in Developmental Disabilities, 32*(6), 2773–2779.
32. Rigoli, D., Piek, J. P., Kane, R., & Oosterlaan, J. (2012). An examination of the relationship between motor coordination and executive functions in adolescents. *Developmental Medicine & Child Neurology, 54*(11), 1025–1031.
33. Efstratopoulou, M., Janssen, R., & Simons, J. (2012). Differentiating children with attention-deficit/hyperactivity disorder, conduct disorder, learning disabilities and autistic spectrum disorders by means of their motor behavior characteristics. *Research in Developmental Disabilities, 33*(1), 196–204.
34. Kadesjo, B., & Gillberg, C. (1999). Developmental coordination disorder in Swedish 7-year-old children. *Journal of the American Academy of Child and Adolescent Psychiatry, 38*(7), 820–828.
35. Schmahmann, J. D. (2004). Disorders of the cerebellum: Ataxia, dysmetria of thought, and the cerebellar cognitive affective syndrome. *The Journal of Neuropsychiatry and Clinical Neurosciences, 16*(3), 367–78.
36. Poore, M. A., & Barlow, S. M. (2009). Suck predicts neuromotor integrity and developmental outcomes. *Perspectives on Speech Science and Orofacial Disorders, 19*(1), 44–51.
37. Francis, D. O., Chinnadurai, S., Morad, A., Epstein, R. A., Kohanim, S., Krishnaswami, S., … McPheeters, M. L. (2015). *Treatments for ankyloglossia and ankyloglossia with concomitant lip-tie* [Internet]. Rockville, MD: Agency for Healthcare Research and Quality (US).

38. Amaizu, N., Shulman, R., Schanler, R., & Lau, C. (2008). Maturation of oral feeding skills in preterm infants.*ActaPaediatrica,97*(1),61–67.Retrievedfromhttp://doi.org/10.1111/j.1651-2227.2007.00548.x
39. Ackermann, H. (2008). Cerebellar contributions to speech production and speech perception: Psycholinguistic and neurobiological perspectives. *Trends in Neurosciences, 31*(6), 265–272.
40. Argyropoulos, G. P. D. (2015). The cerebellum, internal models and prediction in 'non-motor' aspects of language: A critical review. *Brain and Language.* Retrieved from http://dx.doi.org/10.1016/j.bandl.2015.08.003
41. Ainsworth, M. D. S. (1969). Object relations, dependency, and attachment: A theoretical review of the infant-mother relationship. *Child Development, 40*, 969–1025.
42. Shapiro, S. M. (2003). Bilirubin toxicity in the developing nervous system. *Pediatric Neurology, 29*(5), 410–421.
43. Soorani-Lunsing, I., Woltil, H. A., & Hadders-Algra, M. (2001). Are moderate degrees of hyperbilirubinemia in healthy term neonates really safe for the brain? *Pediatric Research, 50*, 701–705.
44. Johnson, L., & Bhutani, V. K. (2011). The clinical syndrome of bilirubin-induced neurologic dysfunction. *Seminars in Perinatology, 35*, 101–113.
45. Shapiro, S. M., & Popelka, G. R. (2011). Auditory impairment in infants at risk for bilirubin-induced neurologic dysfunction. *Seminars in Perinatology, 35*, 162–170.
46. Johnston, M. V., & Hoon, A. H. (2000). Possible mechanisms in infants for selective basal ganglia damage from asphyxia, kernicterus, or mitochondrial encephalopathies. *Journal of Child Neurology, 15*, 588–591.
47. Turkel, S. B. (1990). Autopsy findings associated with neonatal hyperbilirubinemia. *Clinics in Perinatology, 17*, 381–396.
48. Connolly, A. M., & Volpe, J. J. (1990). Clinical features of bilirubin encephalopathy. *Clinics in Perinatology, 17*, 371–379.
49. Rance, G., Beer D. E., Cone-Wesson, B., Shepherd, R. K., Dowell, R. C., King, A. M., … Clark, G. M. (1999). Clinical findings for a group of infants and young children with auditory neuropathy. *Ear and Hearing, 20*, 238–252
50. Vohr, B. R., Karp, D., O'Dea, C., Darrow, D., Coll, C. G., Lester, B. M., … Cashore, W. (1990). Behavioral changes correlated with brain-stem auditory evoked responses in term infants with moderate hyperbilirubinemia. *Journal of Pediatrics, 117*, 288–291.
51. Koziol, L. F., Budding, D. E., & Chidekel, D. (2011). Sensory integration, sensory processing, and sensory modulation disorders: Putative functional neuroanatomic underpinnings. *Cerebellum, 10*(4), 770–792.
52. von Hofsten, C. (2004). An action perspective on motor development. *Trends in Cognitive Sciences, 8*(6), 266–272.
53. von Hofsten, C. (2009). Action, the foundation for cognitive development. *Scandinavian Journal of Psychology, 50*(6), 617–623.
54. Marques, H. G., Bharadwaj, A., & Iida, F. (2014). From spontaneous motor activity to coordinated behaviour: A developmental model. *PLoS Computational Biology, 10*(7), e1003653. doi:10.1371/journal.pcbi.1003653.
55. Strubhar, A. J., Meranda, K., & Morgan, A. (2007). Outcomes of infants with idiopathic hypotonia. *Pediatric Physical Therapy, 19*(3), 227–235.
56. Zoia, S., Blason, L., D'Ottavio, G., Biancotto, M., Bulgheroni, M., & Castiello, U. (2013). The development of upper limb movements: from fetal to post-natal life. *PLoS One, 8*(12), e80876. doi:10.1371/journal.pone.0080876.
57. Futagi, Y., Toribe, Y., & Suzuki, Y. (2012). The grasp reflex and moro reflex in infants: Hierarchy of primitive reflex responses. *International Journal of Pediatrics, 2012*, 191562. doi:10.1155/2012/191562.
58. Moh, W., Graham, J. M., Jr., Wadhawan, I., & Sanchez-Lara, P. A. (2012). Extrinsic factors influencing fetal deformations and intrauterine growth restriction. *Journal of Pregnancy, 2012*, 750485. doi:10.1155/2012/750485.
59. De Jager, M. (2011). *Brain development milestones and learning.* Johannesburg, South Africa: Mind Moves Institute.

60. Winstanley, C. A., Eagle, D. M., & Robbins, T. W. (2006). Behavioral models of impulsivity in relation to ADHD: Translation between clinical and preclinical studies. *Clinical Psychology Review, 26*(4), 379–395. doi:10.1016/j.cpr.2006.01.001.
61. Nayate, A., Bradshaw, J. L., & Rinehart, N. J. (2005). Autism and Asperger's disorder: Are they movement disorders involving the cerebellum and/or basal ganglia? *Brain Research Bulletin, 67*(4), 327–334.
62. Vaidya, C. J. (2012). Neurodevelopmental abnormalities in ADHD. *Current Topics in Behavioral Neurosciences, 9*, 49–66.
63. Roberts, W., Fillmore, M. T., & Milich, R. (2011). Linking impulsivity and inhibitory control using manual and oculomotor response inhibition tasks. *Acta Psychologica, 138*(3), 419–428.
64. Cortese, S., Kelly, C., Chabernaud, C., Proal, E., Di Martino, A., Milham, M. P., & Castellanos, F. X. (2012). Toward systems neuroscience of ADHD: A meta-analysis of 55 fMRI studies. *The American Journal of Psychiatry, 169*(10), 1038–1055
65. Vossel, S., Geng, J. J., & Fink, G. R. (2014). Dorsal and ventral attention systems: Distinct neural circuits but collaborative roles. *The Neuroscientist, 20*(2), 150–159. doi:10.1177/1073858413494269.
66. Persichetti, A. S., Aguirre, G. K., & Thompson-Schill, S. L. (2015). Value is in the eye of the beholder: Early visual cortex codes monetary value of objects during a diverted attention task. *Journal of Cognitive Neuroscience, 27*(5), 893–901. doi:10.1162/jocn_a_00760.
67. Bargh, J., & Uleman, J. S. (1989). *Unintended Thought.* New York, NY: Guilford Publications.
68. Romejko-Wolniewicz, E., Teliga-Czajkowska, J., & Czajkowski, K. (2014). Antenatal steroids: Can we optimize the dose? *Current Opinion in Obstetrics and Gynecology, 26*(2), 77–82. doi:10.1097/GCO.0000000000000047.

Chapter 2
Methods of Neuropsychological Test Interpretation

"I hear and I forget. I see and I remember. I do and I understand."

Confucius

"You cannot create experience. You must undergo it."

Albert Camus

Introduction

This chapter and much of the remaining content of this e-book focuses upon methods of neuropsychological test interpretation. Some graduate students are taught highly specific ways of organizing test data. One method of test interpretation organizes tests according to the domain that corresponds with the name of a test in question. Other students and clinical practitioners simply report test findings by specifically organizing a report according to the name of the test. In our view, this makes the integration of test findings extremely difficult. Reports grounded in this type of framework almost never achieve consistency and seem inherently contradictory. We present a highly specific way of organizing a very high volume of neuropsychological evaluation data. This system avoids all possible interpretative idiosyncrasy, it forces the practitioner to problem-solve when test scores might initially seem contradictory, and it allows the examiner to interpret every case systematically in order to ensure optimal outcomes. Furthermore, this way of interpreting test data leads directly to writing a coherent report, since the data are interpreted in the same way in which the results were initially organized. Therefore, the practitioner never "loses" the original "anchor points." First, we develop a foundation by exploring certain assumptions and facts; this is followed by a systematic interpretative methodology.

© Springer International Publishing Switzerland 2016
L.F. Koziol et al., *Large-Scale Brain Systems and Neuropsychological Testing*,
DOI 10.1007/978-3-319-28222-0_2

Additional Introductory Issues: Assumptions, Facts, and Biases

In our opinion neuropsychological test interpretation is overly reliant upon the transformation of test "behavior" into standard scores. All too often, test publishers force neuropsychological functions into a normal distribution, bell-shaped curve despite the fact that the function being measured may not be normally distributed within the general population [1]. Even when the function being "measured" may not be normally distributed, the function is statistically manipulated, transformed into scaled scores as if the variable in question corresponded to the distribution of a "bell-shaped curve," with the function then categorized in over-arching terms. Summary descriptions such as "high-average", "average", "low-average", etc., reflect whatever category is statistically appropriate. These are merely general terms that do not describe brain-behavior relationships. More often than not, terminologies such as these violate the very definition of clinical neuropsychological evaluation [1]. Categories such as these tell us very little, if anything, about specifying a person's functioning. However, in our experience, there is an overreliance upon this methodology and the subsequent qualification of a given function. In actuality, the distribution of many cognitive functions and behaviors is highly skewed. Some neuropsychological functions are really "have-have not" skills which follow a *dichotomous distribution* [2]. One very obvious function is orientation. You are either oriented to time, place, and person or you are not. Other functions must be individually specified. For instance, having "average executive function" tells us absolutely nothing, but we have read this statement in neuropsychological reports. This chapter was written with this preconceived notion in mind, for the purpose of teaching students of neuropsychology, as well as some practitioners, methodologies for interpreting tests and test scores that will enhance diagnostic accuracy and more directly align neuropsychology with the neurosciences.

In this chapter, the reader will notice that we are merely reemphasizing many of the concepts and ideas previously reviewed by others. For example, composite quotients have little or no place it neuropsychology. Similarly, qualifying terminologies have nothing to do with symptom identification or specifying the nature of brain-behavior relationships. These are critically important points given that neuropsychology seems "stuck" on the idea that summary categorical terms and domain composite scores convey meaningful information about brain functioning. We believe that a test publisher's conversion of all behavioral data into a standard score is simply condescending. It would suggest that neuropsychologists require a simple methodology for understanding brain-behavior relationships. The reality is there is no cookbook methodology for understanding or interpreting neuropsychological data because patient profiles are seldom, if ever, exactly alike.

Exacerbating the issue of brain function standardization are the facts that many test publishers offer computerized test programs, which not only generate the scores, but also computerize and standardize the entire test interpretation. The authors have nothing against using computers to score tests that are cumbersome, and we have nothing against the use of computers to assist with test interpretation. However, we also firmly believe that tests do not render diagnoses. Clinicians make the diagnoses. Determining the diagnosis is the art of our craft and should not be summarized in overarching, "umbrella-like" terms. A computer can assist in scoring tests, it can transform one test score into another type of statistical score for a specific interpretive purpose, and this can provide assistance in assigning meaning to a number. That number might be used as an anchor point for test interpretation. However, it also must be kept in mind that every time a test response is transformed into a number for the purpose of quantification, or for the purpose of the comparison to a group norm, the patient's actual behavior is lost in the score transformation. The behavior is exactly what the neuropsychologist needs to know about and thus the process of standardization may result in missing the forest for the trees. In addition, even average scores may indicate pathology (digits forward and backwards), and should be interpreted within a patient's comprehensive performance throughout an evaluation.

From our point of view, any patient's behavior, and/or any diagnosis, simply cannot be reduced to a set of numbers. In fact, we firmly believe that this type of practice trivializes and diminishes the value of our profession. There is no need for having a doctorate or for a profession called "neuropsychology" if the primary focus is upon quantification, or categorical terms, which say nothing about brain-behavior relationships. Test performances are driven by behavior. We need to know something about the patient's behavior and its relationship to their neuropsychological integrity for the purpose of identifying symptoms or pathology.

An important differentiation needs to be made, and constantly kept in mind, when evaluating a patient. In research settings, there is absolutely no substitute for quantification. However, clinical and experimental studies are conducted on patient populations, usually already diagnosed, and the question becomes how a group of people (usually with certain stratified sample characteristics) with a diagnosis compares to the functioning of a group sample of normal control subjects. Other studies within the spirit of Research Domain Criteria (RDoC) methodology are conducted on a group of individuals with an identified symptom and then compare that symptomatic group to a control population without the given symptom. Other methodologies obviously exist as well. However, *conducting an experimental study is not at all the same as performing a neuropsychological evaluation when a pathology, or symptom, might be expected but has not been formally diagnosed.* So in this way, clinical evaluation can present the neuropsychologist with sort of a "trap." A clinical evaluation is a comprehensive assessment of an "N of 1," instead of evaluating a group "population" and wanting to know how any given individual patient compares to a normal control group *for the purpose of making a diagnosis.* There is nothing wrong with using a score or set of scores to provide a starting point for certain specific interpretations (the subject matter of this book), just so long as the interpreter of the data keeps these distinctions in mind. Using a numeric, statistically derived score is always defined by the interpretive purpose, but there is no single litmus test, or even a pattern of test scores, that generates a specific diagnosis [4, 5], with the possible exception of certain dementia populations [6].

This book is not for the clinical practitioner who believes that "going by the numbers" is the sole method for interpreting test data. We understand that some practitioners believe this is proper practice. We respect that viewpoint. However, we do not agree with that position when the purpose of the assessment is to diagnose pathology or identify symptoms. We adhere to the original definition of neuropsychology as the study of brain-behavior relationships. Furthermore, *quantification in the clinical setting is a sensitive and dangerous policy because "statistical severity" often does not translate to "clinical severity" in an ecologically valid way.* We also know there are plenty of practitioners who are extremely competent and could easily serve as a "model" for illustrating the concepts discussed in this manuscript; for that group, this chapter might not be an appropriate resource. There is considerable variability in the competence of neuropsychological practitioners just as there is variability in any profession. However, if the reader believes that he or she can understand a brain-behavior relationship, make a diagnosis, or identify specific symptoms simply on the basis of numerical data, then their entire notion of neuropsychology is dangerously flawed. Furthermore, we are biased in believing that there have been many advances in the neurosciences over recent years, and that our current knowledge of brain-behavior relationships far surpasses what is usually practiced within traditional clinical neuropsychological evaluation. In fact, there are some aspects of cognition and behavior that cannot be measured or evaluated with existing neuropsychological tests. These points were emphasized in the previous two volumes of this series. There are also numerous "tests" that might even be administered routinely, even though we have no idea as to what might be the neuro-biologic substrate of those tests. Using logical thinking, intuition, and/or tradition does not inform us about how any particular cognitive process is organized within the brain. One of the purposes of this third volume is to bridge the gap between current neuropsychological practice and advances made in other branches of relevant neurosciences. In any case, we are not intending to preach anything to anyone; we admit our biases and the fact that we all write in a direct, blunt fashion that is anything but subtle!

The interpretation of neuropsychological tests, some of which we believe are outmoded, is based upon the practitioner's knowledge of neuroanatomy and subsequent brain behavior relationships. It is also based upon the practitioner's knowledge of how a test was constructed and an understanding of the functional neuroanatomic systems that drive the particular test performance. Depending upon when the reader attended graduate school, this volume might/might not re-hash what the reader previously learned. Within this presentation, we review certain methods of test interpretation that always have been very powerful diagnostically. These methods were once very well known, yet somehow fell out of use in recent decades. In this way, we are not saying anything "new." The remainder of this volume critically analyses contemporary neuropsychological testing and interpretation, questions the utility of neuropsychological tests that are presently in use, discusses multiple methods for interpreting data, and ideally will further facilitate a shift towards developing alternative methodologies for measuring and understanding brain-behavior relationships. We suspect some of these concepts we present will be "new" to many readers.

Collecting Clinical Data: Defining the Problems

An immediate problem that emerges in neuropsychological assessments concerns interpreting tests according to face validity. As can easily be inferred from the first two volumes of this series, the brain does not organize behavior according to the face validity or names of neuropsychological tests. The fact of the matter is that most tests lack face validity. More often than not, any given neuropsychological or cognitive test does not measure only the function that the name of that test implies. Often tests are categorized according to generalized, over-arching "domains" or "categories" despite the fact that the construct presumably measured has no identified neural substrate. One example that immediately comes to mind is the "Auditory Attention and Response Set" subtest of the NEPSY-II [7]. This name implies there is some sort of "pure" domain of "auditory attention." However, this subtest is incredibly dependent upon vision! During task completion, the patient is required to point to various colored shapes. Obviously, this task could never be administered to a blind person since the task requires clear auditory-visual interactions. As a rule of thumb, we believe a test should never be administered and/or interpreted on the basis of face validity or based upon analysis of any categorical, "umbrella" term. And we are in good company, along with authors including Lezak, Howieson, Bigler, & Tranel [1]. There is absolutely no substitute for understanding how a test was constructed, learning about the specific skills that are required in order to perform on any given test, and then determining what brain systems or networks are engaged when an individual is completing the particular test. And we do not know the neuro-biologic substrates of many tests. When that level or degree of understanding is appreciated and achieved, it becomes "safe" and clinically meaningful to both administer and interpret a test or group of tests. And many of these variables might never be known, as is the case for many subtests of the Wechsler Intelligence Scales for Children, Fifth Edition and its earlier editions [8]. This statement extends to include the adult versions as well. Then again, this group of subtests never were intended to be applied as neuropsychological tests.

To serve as other examples, the Wisconsin Card Sort Test, the Tower of London test, and the Tower of Hanoi are often all considered frontal lobe tests and tests of one's executive functioning. However, the fact of the matter is that intra-individual performances on these three tests have a very low correlation coefficient. This literally means that these three executive function tests cannot possibly be measuring the same abstract construct, cognition, or behavior. As reviewed in *Subcortical Structures and Cognition* [9], each of these three tests activates different brain regions during the course of test performance. Therefore, it must be concluded that these three tests all measure different aspects of brain-behavior relationships. Similarly, while many constructs seem to be understood as static entities, in actuality, test performances are typically dynamic, recruiting different brain regions as task performance progresses or unfolds. This makes good sense in view of the findings of Cole and colleagues [10, 11]. In studying the fronto-parietal network (FPN), they found that novel tasks dependent upon cognitive control always recruited a unique set of brain regions in addition to the FPN; in other words, the

FPN was considered a "flexible hub" that activated whatever brain regions were necessary to complete any given task. Numerous other examples can be given. The studies by Cole's group of investigators used 64 separate tasks. However, the fact of the matter is that this "multiple brain region" task network "principle" is true of just about every specific test for any "domain" in clinical neuropsychology which is one reason why artificially, conceptually or theoretically defined domain analysis is misleading.

It is well known and accepted in neuroscience that the needs of human interactive behavior require continuous neural processing. This neural processing occurs within large scale brain systems as discussed in volumes I and II of this series. These brain networks process or "code" the salient, relevant properties of objects, such as what they look like and feel like, as well as what they are used for and how to use them. All experiences, including *interactions with neuropsychological tests,* are represented or retained in the same sensory and motor brain networks and circuits that were activated, or recruited, when the "information" about the experiences was initially acquired [12–17]. With respect to the current "executive function domain" under discussion, the "bullet point" to keep in mind is that activities, choices, or decisions are represented over large regions of the brain and that this is a process of dynamic interaction and not a static entity. These functions are not specifically localized within the prefrontal cortex or the FPN; they are localized within the same sensory and motor circuits that were activated when first "processing" that information. These neuroscientific "facts" (which we prefer to call interim theoretical solutions) undermine theoretical "umbrella term" constructs such as executive function, language, attention, etc., because we now need to think about these global categorical constructs in a different way. On the other hand, it explains phenomenon every clinical practitioner has observed, including "failures" in performances on neuropsychological tests against the background of adaptive "real life" adjustment. It also explains the opposite, such as good neuropsychological test performance with poor "real life" executive functioning. We can understand that a "central executive" has never been found or located within the brain because there is none! (see volumes I and II of this series for important reviews.) Just as adaptation depends upon ongoing interactions with the environment, an evaluation requires changing, ongoing interactions with neuropsychological tests. Unfortunately, very many neuropsychological tests are outdated and likely do not measure what they purport to measure. Unfortunately, we are applying certain tests without knowing their underpinnings [18]. The interested reader who is unfamiliar with this concept, or the reader who wishes to explore this concept further, is referred to *Subcortical Structures and Cognition* [9], *The Neuropsychological Evaluation of the Child* [19], and/or *Neuropsychological Testing* [1]. *The Compendium of Neuropsychological Tests* [20] can also be quite useful in finding explanations related to test administration and measurement, if the test measures the function in question, and what actual neuropsychological underpinnings the test might be assessing. Therefore, the clinical practitioner has a number of resources at his or her disposal in order to obtain at least some basic insights concerning the variables involved in test construction and performance.

Another issue that needs to be addressed concerns the problem of test revision and recency. What are misunderstood as ethical mandates, and perhaps a lack of reflection over what processes and functions an examiner is attempting to measure, nearly force practitioners to use the most recent version of a test. However, test revision does not guarantee that the revised version of the test will measure the same function as the previous version. In many instances, knowing whether or not the test measures the same function after it has been revised involves knowing the correlation between the two different versions of the test. If the correlation coefficient is relatively low, the practitioner should have the option of determining whether or not the use of the new version is clinically indicated or sound. A close examination of the newer test and the older test should be undertaken. In clinical neuropsychology, "new" is not synonymous with "better".

We propose there are a variety of tests that simply never need to be revised. For example, tests that evaluate pathognomonic or specific signs of impairment are tests that do not require revision. For instance, it might be useful for the practitioner to ask himself or herself whether or not the neurologist's finger-to-nose test was ever revised. The fact of the matter is that this test has specific pathognomonic significance. Each and every time a positive behavior is observed the finding is relevant clinically. The test never needs revision because it measures a very basic but critical function, and the interpretation of the meaning of that test is the same each and every time. This would provide another salient example of how a test could be forced into a standardized, normative distribution, or perhaps some other score; however, this would lead to a misleading interpretation. The test is one of pathognomonic significance with standardization being irrelevant and unnecessary. There are certain specific or pathognomonic signs of impairment in neuropsychological assessment as well, and these tests never really need revision. However, in order to make this determination as to whether a test/procedure is of pathognomonic significance, the practitioner needs to understand the neurobiologic substrate of that particular behavior. In the case of this particular example, we are evaluating the presence or absence of a cerebellar control model [21].

Other tests tend to be more dependent upon cultural factors. Many of these tests require revision from time to time, in order to stay abreast of cultural or social changes. Tests such as these are often uninformative in neuropsychological assessment. However, this is certainly not the case for every test that is used in neuropsychology, regardless of the normative standardization sample upon which the test was initially constructed. Similarly, the authors are well aware that American Psychological Association's Ethical Principles require the practitioner to use the most recent version of tests. However, our ethics code also has a provision allowing the use of dynamic batteries. The code allows the use of tests deemed clinically relevant and justifiable. If the clinician is forced to use current or updated measures routinely, without clinical judgment, then neuropsychology is not in control of its own profession.

Inherent in our concern about test revision is the fact that too often the updated version of the test does not align with our current understanding about brain-behavior relationships. The revision is not initiated based upon what we have learned about the organization of behavior within the brain; rather the test is simply being "updated" with respect to the outcomes obtained by a more current population. There are some tests and methodologies that have been well researched. Therefore, numerous aspects of these tests and test batteries might not require any revision whatsoever. In these cases rigidly adhering to a principle of using the newest test version may place the practitioner in the position of using a test that is poorly researched, poorly constructed, and has limited or no empirical support related to what the test purports to measure. We hope to make the practitioner aware that there is considerable leeway in test-choice during an evaluation, and that decisions should be made on the basis of whether or not the test in question measures what it actually is supposed to measure. This requires the examiner's clinical judgment. However, clinical judgment is not the same as "hunch" or intuition. Perhaps as a general rule, if the examiner can put into words what he or she wants to measure, and describe the accepted substrate of the behavior and how the test measures it, then the clinician is relying upon judgment; if that "judgment" is reduced to "hunch," there is likely an issue of clinical understanding. Furthermore, we want to emphasize the point that certain skills are amenable to quantification while other functions are not amenable to quantification and standardization methodologies. For example, consider the case below:

Case 4: Timmy

A late aged toddler sustained a documented anoxic brain injury secondary to ingesting approximately 100 mg of a toxic substance that coated a pellet painting toy of the time. The child became anoxic and went into a coma for 24 hours. Medical professionals told the parents that the child was fine upon coming out of the coma. However, the parents noticed the child did not have near the vocabulary he previously had, the left corner of his mouth slightly drooped and he was constantly sucking that part of the lip into his mouth. An additional symptom concerned the child's lack of pain or taste reception in his mouth. The child could eat piping hot French fries without wincing and would burn his mouth. He also could run barefoot on small pebbles without feeling pain. He began playing with his feces which was hard and pebble like. As the child grew, he threw temper tantrums, exhibited motor and speech apraxia and what seemed like ADHD with severe impulsivity.

The child also showed a complete loss of smell and severe sinus complications. In fact, he could not register that his sinuses were full in order to prompt him to blow his nose, which his parents reported he was previously able to notice and try to do. The impacted sinuses and drainage caused sleep disturbance, and many sinus and lung infections. The child was nearly constantly prescribed antibiotics.

By 4 years old the child was toilet trained for bladder but not bowel. In fact, by 10 years old the child never attained bowel control. The curse of his brain injury is that he cannot control his bowels and he cannot smell when he has had an accident, which then generates a severe emotional reaction.

Several medical disciplines including neurology, developmental pediatrics, gastroenterology, and allergists evaluated the child. He also was evaluated by specialists in neuropsychology, speech/language pathology, and occupational and physical therapists. It was generally agreed that the child was experiencing deficits in attention and executive functioning (albeit in an atypical manner), apraxia, oral motor and sensory issues, and learning disabilities. In this regard, the neuropsychological test data were not informative in addressing the child's presenting problems.

The case became a civil suit and the toy company's experts indicated the child was suffering from allergies, behavioral bowel retention, autism, oppositional defiant disorder, and parental hospitalization syndrome (despite a 24 hour hospitalization). In other words, the defense professionals blamed the child and the parents for his way of being.

Upon further medical and neuropsychological evaluation, allergies and autism were correctly ruled out. A gastroenterology note remarked that the child had impacted bowel, but no pain. Finally, as part of a neuropsychology evaluation, the defense psychologist wrote that the Romberg test and Finger-Nose were administered and the results were *positive*, but this person did not elaborate about what that meant. The Romberg test has the examinee stand with legs together, eyes closed, and arms outstretched. The clinician pushes down on the arms. A positive finding means the person could not sustain their balance. Positive findings on these screening tests implicate abnormalities in subcortical functions, possibly including brainstem, cortico-striatal, and cerebro-cerebellar systems.

Brain injury was successfully argued by the plaintiff's neuropsychologist, without doing further neuropsychological evaluation. The impacted bowel along with no pain secondary to colon stretching is significant. The colon only has stretch receptors for pain [22]; therefore, the ascending sensory stimulus was not being registered by the brain. This points to CNS "brain-related involvement" and not peripheral spinal damage. Intact, urinary continence (an anterior neuronal process) with impaired bowel continence implicates the pudendal nerve (a posterior localized brain function), which also communicates ascending sensory information to the brain [23]. The lack of pain in the feet, further implicates reception of ascending sensory stimulus to the brain. All of these ascending fibers communicate through the gracillis fasciculus and lemniscus, which also is innervated by the brain stem/cerebellum. These tracts finally terminate in the posterior ventral thalamus before registering in the sensory cortex. Again, this means that the brain is not registering certain, localized sensory information.

Similarly, the sinus problems, lack of smell, apraxia, left mouth droop, lack of oral pain and poor oral motor control implicate the trigeminal and olfactory nerves. The trigeminal and olfactory nerves form the trigeminal-thalamic pathway that terminates in the posterior ventral thalamus [24].

In this case, neuropsychological test results were confounding and not what one would expect because they do not evaluate regions of the brain that appear to be the most heavily involved in the pathology. Therefore, a "number driven" evaluation would lead an examiner astray towards a false negative finding. Perhaps the erroneous assumption was made that ability and behavioral control are always under voluntary control and perhaps only cortically-driven. There is no relevant way to quantify this behavior.

The Quantification of Behavior

A simple exercise enables us to illustrate a basic point. We have chosen the Wechsler Scales, although almost any cognitive and/or neuropsychological test can be used for this particular purpose. The reader can choose any one of the Wechsler IQ scales, any version whatsoever, from the initial Wechsler-Bellevue scale, up until the present time. However, since other tests are scored in a similar fashion, and since most examiners administer intelligence tests in a standard "battery" (often Wechsler Scales), this seems to be a particularly easy place to start.

How are the Wechsler scales actually scored? Let us simply run through the process. First, after the individual takes the examination, every individual item is scored. Every single response is converted to a score, either a zero, one, or two-point response, whatever the case may be for any particular subtest. Second, this is done for each and every item within each subtest. Third, scores are then aggregated on every subtest. Fourth, the aggregate raw score is then converted to a scaled score. Fifth, this process is performed on each and every subtest for every "Index" that is administered for the scale. Sixth, after summarizing these subtests, the subtest's scaled scores are then aggregated to obtain the composite quotient. The point we are trying to make is simple. By the time the final score is calculated, that particular score is at least six times removed the from the patient's original reply. The questions we pose are these: What does this score actually mean if it is removed at least six times from the patient's original response? What is wrong with the patient's original response to begin with? Why are so many conversions required to "understand" the behavior?

Obviously, there are no answers to these questions, other than for serving the purpose of statistical manipulation for standardization. Similarly, we are not criticizing the process. We are merely asking the clinical examiner to think about what he or she is doing during the process of test scoring and test interpretation. It is certainly true that in order to obtain quantification, some sort of conversion process is required. This enables us to compare a numerical performance with a numerical, statistical normative standard. However, we are also asking the examiner to consciously be aware of the fact that the numeric values obtained are far removed from the patient's original product *and that in this process of data collection, the clinical information we are most interested in is lost.* The clinical examiner simply must return to where the patient started in order to achieve any real interpretive value from this process or to derive meaning from any possible quantification. In addition, there are obvious characteristics about a patient's response that can never be quantified, while these aspects of what the patient said or did can never achieve meaning by assigning the original response products to a numeric value. In this way, it seems easy for us to defend our position that a competent clinical neuropsychologist can never evaluate any individual patient by simply "going by the numbers." The patient's behavior has meaning. This meaning informs us about possible brain-behavior relationships. Quantification is absolutely necessary for experimental investigations. However, every neuropsychological evaluation is an "N of 1."

We illustrate these comments with the adult version of the Wechsler Working Memory Index (WMI) which includes the Arithmetic and Digit Span (DS) tests. First, the Arithmetic test is only a working memory task if the patient does not have dyscalculia or problems with attention, impulsivity, and receptive language, which are but a few confounds that can lower scores on this test. The task is overly multi-factorial to be considered a pure measure of working memory. Second, the Digit Span tasks are fraught with problems. DS is two subtests that most clinicians report with one score. Digits Forward is an encoding task, while Digits Backward might be considered an explicit working memory task. Let's consider a hypothetical example; a person performs at the 75th percentile on Digits Forward and the 5th percentile on the Digits Backwards task. The DS score will be at about the 25th percentile and the clinician will no doubt state the individual does not have a working memory deficit as measured by a subtest that considers working memory a static, blatantly explicit function; after all it is an average score under the WMI. The clinician must evaluate error variance. For example, a 7 year old child who correctly encodes and recalls six digits twice across two trials is performing well. But what if the same child recalled five, four, and three digits once across two trials each? The score would be lower, but only the clinician who reviews the protocol to see the variance will understand that the capacity for encoding is large, but the outcome score is poor secondary to the child's apparent inattentiveness or distractibility during trials. In any case, for some reason, the performance is highly variable, which is the critical conclusion to be inferred. The same can be said for Digits Backwards. An additional thought on DS has to do with the person who performs better on the more difficult Digits Backwards task than the easier Digits Forward task. As a rule of thumb, the score on Digits Forward should always be higher than it is on Digits Backwards. The score for DS would be misleading and likely incorrectly interpreted. This case represents the 'have/have' not nature of aspects of attention systems. No one is completely without attention. Attention is variably expressed and will randomly undermine the full expression of otherwise intact encoding and working memory capacity. Therefore, a child, or adult, may perform better on a more difficult task than a similar but easier task. In the absence of a qualitative review of testing performance one may misattribute this kind of testing outcome as a lack of effort on the part of the patient. If variability is truly a test performance outcome on the basis of the nature of attention, then our conclusions are plausible; if an examiner believes every test performance represents the person's "best effort," then the results are uninterpretable; *any time a test performance can be interpreted more than one way, our inclination is to view that data as "uninterpretable."*

Levels of Inference in Neuropsychological Test Interpretation

Neuropsychological evaluations generate a voluminous amount of data. The primary problem with obtaining this volume of results concerns ways to organize this information for the purpose of appropriate interpretation. Perhaps Hallstead and

Retain were among the first to propose a methodology for data organization. The organizational methodology which they developed is certainly not restricted to the Halstead-Retain battery. In our own opinion, this particular methodology for organizing data might represent their greatest contribution in terms of testing in the field of neuropsychology. The fact that this methodology is certainly not unique to the Hallstead-Retain battery, and has been comprehensively described by other well known authors, chief of which are Lezak [1] and Baron [19], attests to its broad-based applications. We believe the aforementioned texts should be standard reading for anyone who practices clinical and/or pediatric neuropsychology. In addition to providing organization of the data, this methodology allows for a systematic interpretation of test results. It enables the examiner to not only manage a large volume of information, but it also allows the examiner to review every case, in exactly the same way, each and every time a clinical case is interpreted. Four levels of inferential analysis were proposed.

The Level of Performance

The first method for analyzing neuropsychological test results concerns the simple level of performance criteria. This is literally the most basic way for attributing meaning to quantified test results. In this methodology, an individual's test score is compared to an objective normative standard. That objective normative standard is usually a normally distributed bell-shaped curve. At this basic level, there are only three possible outcomes. First, a poor level of performance usually implies some sort of impairment in each and every instance. However, the most critically important point concerning a poor level of performance is the fact that at this level of analysis, the reason for the poor performance level can never be identified. Using this methodology, we ultimately know that any given subject's test performance is below expectation relative to a group standard, with the important caveats that the skills in question are normally distributed, in other words, following the normal distribution of a bell-shaped curve. So, at this level, if, for example, a patient's score is a standard deviation below the mean, we can identify that score as falling at the 16th percentile ranking, as being poorer than expected, or "Below Average," without knowing anything about the reason this low performance occurred. If the patient's level of performance falls two standard deviations below average, the only thing we really know is that this patient performed very poorly, within the "Impaired" range, but once again, the specific reason as to why that performance was so far below expectation remains unknown.

Another outcome might be that the patient's level of performance falls right in the middle of the expected range. At this level, a score is usually termed "Average." However, once again, the reason for this level of performance is not known. Other outcomes include scores a standard deviation above the mean, typically termed "Above Average," or two standard deviations above the mean, typically referred to as "Very Superior," and so on and so forth. However, to reiterate, the reason for the good performance is not known. These are the problems inherent in constantly referring to the normal distribution of a bell-shaped curve, as well as the problems within terminologies, which are categorical such as "average." Therefore, quantification and categorization of functioning may be of limited clinical utility even when measuring functions that are normally distributed.

Comparing a subject to any normally distributed group norm tells you absolutely nothing about the patient in question, other than how that person performed relative to a recognized group standard. Similarly, comparing an individual's performance indiscriminately to the patient's test scores on other tasks may result in inaccurate assumptions and misdiagnoses. Intra-individual comparison requires an examiner to make assumptions, which might or might not be true. This may increase the likelihood of making false positive and/or false negative errors. For example, an examiner may compare a patient's level of performance on an intelligence test to a level of performance on another test, a practice which is technically referred to as "cognitive referencing."[25]. *Unless the relationship between two test scores is known*, then simply put, those two independent test performances should not be compared. All test results should be interpreted in an objective, systematic, non-idiosyncratic fashion. One examiner may not be interpreting data using the same set of assumptions as another examiner, which leads two examiners to interpret the same outcomes in very different ways.

Pattern Analysis

The second the level of inferential analysis concerns test score comparisons that is sometimes referred to as "pattern analysis." A comparison of test scores often generates synergistic patterns of functioning that would not be available through simply interpreting test scores in isolation. However, it is critical to understand that in order to use this type of methodology a comprehensive understanding of what the test is measuring is essential. For example, one simple comparison concerns relating a score on a semantic/category fluency subtest to a score on a letter or phonemic fluency subtest. It is known that the brain stores information according to semantic categories. Therefore, this is a reliable way for understanding performance on category fluency subtests, since language is understood as a semantic classification system. Language evolved for many reasons, but one reason was to make sense out of or categorize complex sensory stimuli. An efficient and economical method of organization is to place various sensory stimuli into semantic categories. Semantic categories immediately tell an individual how objects might be alike, and how they simultaneously might be different. This is essential for survival.

Inherent in the semantic classification system is the ventral attention network, which stores names of objects according to their meaning or "worth." In other words, the brain naturally stores information according to semantic properties, which are meaningful for adaptation or survival. On the other hand, letter fluency, sometimes referred to as phonemic fluency, has nothing to do with the manner in which the brain retains information.

Letter or phonemic fluency tasks require an individual to retrieve words having little to do with the word's meaning or the way words are naturally stored within the brain. Retrieval of words based upon the initial starting letter mitigates the efficiency of the brain's innate information retention system. The brain simply does not store information like a dictionary, ranging from the letters A to Z. Therefore, comparing performances on these two subtests becomes meaningful. In this regard, both semantic/category fluency and letter/phonemic fluency require recruitment of the exact same retrieval mechanism, specifically, a frontal-striatal circuitry that governs language production. In this regard, when comparing performance on a category fluency task with performance on a letter fluency task only three outcomes are possible. First, performances on both tasks can be significantly depressed. Since both tasks require the same retrieval mechanism, this pattern might be interpreted as reflecting a language-related disorder, specifically, a deficit in word retrieval. Alternatively, this finding can be a manifestation of a poorly developed vocabulary. Second, semantic fluency can be depressed relative to the performance on a letter fluency task. This type of pattern is frequently observed in early onset alzheimer's disease patients [6]. In Alzheimer's disease, semantic networks literally deteriorate. Therefore, a poor performance on a semantic fluency task relative to a preserved performance on a letter fluency subtest might reflect a deterioration in the brain's semantic networks. A third possible outcome concerns good category/semantic fluency performance relative to poor performance on letter fluency tests. Since we already know that both subtests share the same retrieval mechanism, the difference in test scores cannot possibly be due to a retrieval issue. At the same time, since we know the brain stores information according to semantic networks, we immediately know that the good semantic fluency performance must be a manifestation of intact semantic networks. Those with depressed phonemic language retrieval are likely demonstrating functional impairment in an anterior brain region. Retrieving words according to the starting letter requires the individual to develop his or her own retrieval strategy in order to be appropriately efficient in retrieving words. This type of strategy development is exactly what is missing from performance on a semantic fluency task, which allows the patient to rely upon the natural organization of the structure of language. In this way, by comparing the proper subtest scores, which can only occur when we understand the underpinnings of the tasks in question, our interpretation becomes a synergistic one. This allows the examiner to identify possible deficits, learning something new about the patient in question that we would never have known if we relied simply upon a level of performance criteria. By combining the appropriate data, our interpretation has become synergistic. We have placed ourselves within an interpretive paradigm that allows us to focus upon symptom identification.

Pathognomonic Signs

The third level of inferential analysis refers to specific or pathognomonic signs. This level might be understood as a specific instance of a level of performance criteria. However, in this case, "level of performance" has nothing to do with the normal distribution of a bell-shaped curve. Instead, pathognomonic signs represent highly specific behaviors that point to specific pathology in each and every instance in which these signs are observed. Pathognomonic signs are dichotomous in distribution. For example, the neurologist employs the finger-to-nose test as a pathognomonic sign approach. The results of this simple test revealed to the neurologist whether or not the cerebellum is capable of adapting to the changing requirements of movement as the simple task unfolds. In a sense, this is a highly specific instance of a "level of performance" approach to interpretation. However, it does not follow the normal distribution of a bell-shaped curve. Instead, this is literally a "have" or "have not" level of performance criteria.

In neuropsychology, there are numerous pathognomonic signs. For example, disorientation to time, place, and person are all specific signs of brain impairment. Disorientation to time tells us that the patient is no longer capable of registering experience in time, in an ongoing way. The finding always carries the exact same interpretation. If a child has had appropriate exposure to educational curriculum at a certain point a spelling error that deviates from the phonological properties of the intended word represents a pathognomonic sign related to one's understanding of sound-letter correspondences. Sometimes called a "dysphonetic" spelling error, the mistake which illustrates the patient cannot make a word "look" the way it "sounds" is highly specific to a learning disorder which typically includes both spelling and reading [26]. Another pathognomonic sign might be understood as representing a rule violation on a test like the Tower of London test. There are basic rules to follow in the performance of this problem-solving subtest, and in each and every instance when a task-rule violation occurs, it represents a failure of thought to guide problem-solving behavior. This is a specific sign of cognitive impairment typically reflecting inhibitory deficits, often indicative of "stimulus-bound" behavior. Other signs of pathognomonic significance include commission errors on *certain types* of stop signal tasks, go-no go tasks, or continuous performance tasks. However, once again, when using tasks to evaluate specific or pathognomonic signs, it becomes critical to understand the underlying structure of how the test was constructed and its neurobiologic substrate, particularly since the interpretation automatically points to significant pathological behavior.

The Analysis of Sensory and Motor Data

The fourth level of inference for analyzing neuropsychological data was originally introduced as body side comparisons. Sensory and motor data were obtained for both sides of the body on a variety of measures and comparisons were made between functioning of the dominant hand and functioning on the non-dominant hand. The HRB includes the motor tasks finger tapping and grip strength. Sensory tasks included finger localization/discrimination and tests of agnosia, which required the subject to identify objects simply by touch. The original finger tapping tasks and grip strength tests represented very limited samples of motor functioning, restricted to just a few ventral brain regions. Sensory tasks were also limited in the sense that agnosia and finger localization were the primary tasks evaluated. This method of analysis remains appropriate. For example, on motor tasks a right-hand dominant patient is expected to perform at a level 10 % greater than their performance with the non-dominant left hand. The opposite relationship was expected in a left-hand dominant person. On sensory tasks, equal performances were expected bilaterally.

Most examiners consider an examination of sensory-motor systems as optional in today's neuropsychological evaluation. However, in our position, it is absolutely critical to evaluate motor behavior, and this becomes particularly necessary with respect to the evaluation of the pediatric patient population. The motor system is believed to achieve maturity somewhere between the ages of 10 and 12 years of age [27, 28]. Within this age range, the motor system should be considered stable and adult level performances should be expected by the time the child reaches 12 years old. However, in the current state of our knowledge, and the relationship between movement and thought which has been emphasized elsewhere of this series [29], we believe it is absolutely critical to include an extensive sensory and motor examination in all neuropsychological assessments. The reason for this position is obvious; motor behavior and control over the motor system represents the forerunner of cognitive development or executive and/or cognitive control. With respect to the adult population, Goldberg and Podel, et al., have described a systematic evaluation of sensory and motor functioning in the Executive Control Battery [30]. This is essentially the same examination that was developed by Luria in order to systematically evaluate the motor system. With respect to child populations, numerous evaluations are commercially available. Martha Denkla has developed the PANNES [31], which represents a simple, yet systematic evaluation of certain motor functions, of pathognomonic significance, that later support higher-level cognitive functions. Similarly, certain versions of the NEPSY include a reasonably systematic assessment of sensory and motor behavior. The critical importance of these examinations was described in *The Myth of Executive Functioning* [4].

A 10 % difference between dominant and non-dominant hands obviously cannot be identified in a highly systematic motor examination that includes the acquisition of new, coordinated bi-manual movements. These aspects of the systematic assessment require bilateral motor programming, and one would certainly not expect to measure a difference in functioning between the dominant and non-dominant hands on these types of tasks. Instead, these tasks should be interpreted in more of a pathognomonic fashion, particularly since the motor system matures relatively early, with motor development representing the ongoing development of the substrate of cognitive control. In fact, it can be stated that a young child's primary "job" during the course of development is to master control over the motor system, since motor control is critical as we interact within a constantly changing environment. Similarly, numerous studies have demonstrated the intrinsic and intricate relationship between the integrity of the motor system and a variety of neuro- developmental disorders that typically persist well into adulthood although the symptomatic picture often changes. In any case, the most critical factor being emphasized concerns the necessity of a systematic evaluation of motor and sensory functions. Motor and sensory systems should be evaluated individually, and other tasks should be included that require sensory-motor integrative functions. Motor tasks can never be "pure." However, tests have been developed that emphasize either motor or sensory functioning individually, while other tests exist that integrate both sensory and motor behaviors. The following case vignette illustrates a variety of important variables:

This child was 11 years old at the time of this evaluation. She was diagnosed with Gomez-Lopez-Hernandez Syndrome, a very rare disorder of the cerebellum. We will refer to this case in the following chapters to illustrate other features of her functioning relevant to the interpretation of neuropsychological tests. She obtained the following scores on the "Sensorimotor Functions" domain of the NEPSY:

Subtest	Scaled score/Percentile rank
Fingertip tapping	12
Imitating hand positions	7
Visuomotor precision	4
Manual motor sequencing	3rd–10th percentile
Finger discrimination preferred right hand	50th–75th percentile
Finger discrimination non-preferred hand	50th–75th percentile

The NEPSY combines sensory and motor functioning into a unitary domain. Therefore, certain test scores need to be disambiguated. Sensory-perceptual functions are intact as measured by finger localization behavior. These functions should provide support for imitating hand positions. The poor performance on the imitating hand positions subtest is likely the introduction of the motor component. Nevertheless, since this subtest combines the performances of both hands, the "raw score" data need to be examined. In this case, the right hand performance was a raw score of 10; the left hand raw score was 11. These are equivalent scores, implying equal functioning on both body sides. The child made very few errors, since 12 raw score "points" is the maximum. This means it is extremely rare to see a child of her age functioning that poorly; the subtest tolerates little error so that these performances might be considered pathognomonic of the symptom of "dyspraxia." Impulsive responses were observed on the beginning easier items. On difficult items, she used her "other hand" to complete accurate modeling of the hand positions; this must mean that "visual" sensory input was intact because she observed the stimulus positions accurately. This implies difficulty with finger dexterity, primarily a motor component. On one item that required her to imitate the position of forming the hand and fingers to resemble a "telephone," the modeling of the position was correct; however, she "missed her mouth," regardless of body side. Therefore, in addition to the limited interpretation provided by "numbers," considerable clinical information emerged from observing the quality of her behaviors. The additional interpretative features include the emphasis on motor output instead of sensory input, as well as the "over-shooting, undershooting" of missing the mouth, implying the dysmetria often observed in patients with a compromised cerebellar control model.

The motor task performances are similarly informative. At first glance, fingertip tapping looks like a very impressive scaled score! However, performances were always very fast and accompanied by an inability to maintain the proper finger tapping and finger sequencing positions. The "pincer finger grasp," often indicative of the integrity of cerebellar control, was actually absent; in this way, an initially impressive looking score is significantly degraded, while observational data lead to useful interpretation. In addition, the score on the visuomotor precision subtest in decidedly poor. The tasks were performed impulsively, and so quickly that no subject could have performed accurately. It appeared as though she misjudged the difficulty of the task, which is equivalent to interpreting a lack of control over the motor system; this often corresponds to a more generalized lack of self-regulation. In addition, her pencil grip was anomalous; she held the pencil between her third and fourth fingers while placing her thumb over all fingers; this compromised fine motor control since she controlled the pencil with whole arm movements. This implies a lack of development from proximal to distal motor regions, with the exact same interpretation of poor control over the motor system. Finally, on the series of motor sequencing tasks, most motor "programs" were intact, but there were so many significant observations that "raw scores" were subjectively degraded. For instance, rhythmic timing was virtually absent; the "force" of movement was often excessive, reflecting a type of "hypermetric" behavior, similar to the concept of "over-shooting" mentioned above; test items requiring bimanual wrist coordination were all performed with whole arm movements, which again suggested adequate "programming" but deficient motor development. There was considerable "associated movement," often termed "motor overflow," observed by her involuntary mouth and tongue movements. Uncontrolled, "rolling" head movements were observed throughout the course of administration of all tasks within this generalized NEPSY domain (which is characteristic of the pathology described in future chapters).

In summary, systematic interpretation of these data reveals many of the points made in the aforementioned text. The limitations of scaled and raw scores were illustrated; the element of subjectivity was illustrated in terms of scoring behavioral observations. The necessity for disambiguating "combined domain" scores was demonstrated. An example of inferring motor development, or lack thereof, was implicated; it was further demonstrated that how behavioral observations can be applied to inform test interpretation and localization, in this case, emphasizing the role of the cerebellum in controlling the force, rate and rhythm of behavior. In view of the fact that it is generally accepted knowledge by now that motor system development is complete, reaching adult levels of performance between the ages of 10–12 years, the findings take on pathognomonic significance. Finally, the child's behaviors were consistent with expectations as described in *ADHD as a Model of Brain-Behavior Relationships* [3] and *The Myth of Executive Functioning* [4].

Interim Summary

We have indicated that most neuropsychological evaluations include a volume of data. It is critically important to evaluate that data in a systematic manner. Therefore, the first step in approaching data analysis requires an in depth understanding of the neurobiologic substrates of sensory-perceptual and motor or action systems, or how these systems are organized within the brain. We have presented a system for organizing neuropsychological data that allows the examiner to interpret data in the same way, every single time, for every case that he or she evaluates. This system should be applied so routinely that it eventually becomes implicit in the examiner's way of both gathering and interpreting test results. Similarly, aspects of this organizational system can be applied to every traditional domain within neuropsychological assessment. For instance, it is extremely clear that the level of performance criteria, test score comparisons, and the identification of pathognomonic signs can be applied to the domains of language, attention, executive functioning, visual-spatial functioning, and even learning and memory. The sensory and motor evaluations represent their own separate "domains", although it is clear that these functions support each and every other domain of cognitive functioning. Similarly, it is always important to recognize the artificiality of "domains," which is not to say neuropsychological test results cannot be organized within a domain structure as an initial step for test interpretation.

Challenges for Neuropsychology

Above we described how neuropsychological domains were artificially derived. When the field of neuropsychology was in its infancy it may have made sense to separate various cognitive functions into domains to standardize the interpretive process, even though there was limited neuroanatomic functional data to support the existence of explicit domains. However, we now know that in neuroscience there is not an isolated and dedicated system that is specific to language functioning. Instead, we find the FPN recruits multiple regions to support language comprehension and expression. In addition, there is simply no circuitry that is solely dedicated to any specific "domain". There is no specific domain of attention. Executive functions such as planning and organization are not located in a single distinct area and in fact require the recruitment of multiple systems. The same holds true for any other domain. Even sensory-motor tasks may recruit brain regions outside of the sensory-motor system depending upon the task in question. In short, all cognitive functioning is clearly both localized and distributed. As nicely summarized by a number of researchers, cognition and behavior are stored or retained in the exact same regions that were activated when those experiences originally occurred [32]. We are suggesting that perhaps this requires a paradigm shift in the way we ultimately understand neuropsychological test results. Similarly, as has been reviewed comprehensively in other manuscripts, the brain simply does not organize behavior on the basis of verbal versus non-verbal function. Instead, brain-behavior relationships appear to be organized with respect to a novelty-routinization principle. We typically function in routine circumstances.

On occasion, we function under novel circumstances. These conditions require us to problem-solve, and once the problem is solved, and the more we engage in that particular behavior, the more automatic that behavior becomes. In other words, the human brain functions in an extremely economical fashion, typically automatically, with the ultimate goal of functioning being to take that which is novel and make the behavior automatic with repeated exposure and practice. Behaviors that are independent of conscious cognitive control are much more economical since they conserve valuable cognitive resources and energy. Conservation of resources was emphasized in *The Myth of Executive Functioning* [4]. In our opinion, test interpretation needs to be organized and modified accordingly. In subsequent chapters, we will demonstrate how by changing certain methods of test administration, neuropsychological evaluation can be modified to reflect this operational novelty-routinization principle.

A paradigm shift actually represents an extremely significant challenge for clinical neuropsychology. For example, the evidence is extremely persuasive that there is no specific "domain" for anything [33]. Instead, we find activation of a cognitive control system that recruits other brain regions that are necessary for the completion of any particular task in question. There is not one "attention" system. Instead, there is a ventral attention network that assigns meaning to circumstances and a dorsal attention network that allows us to interact with the environment as circumstances change [34]. In this way, there is a close interplay between the ventral and dorsal attention networks, and an individual's capacity for cognitive control, which is presumably governed by the bi-laterally distributed FPNs. We find a default mode network that allows us to rely on past experiences for planning, organization, thinking and problem-solving, again interacting with FPNs. Instead of finding a compartmentalized "emotional" network, we find a limbic network that closely interacts with other brain networks, including the ventral attention network in order to provide salience to situations and to provide appropriate motivation for reward-based learning. We find that there are no separate visual and auditory attention systems [35]. Instead, we find that attention networks are actually anchored in the heart of the visual network, which supports both object identification and localization for appropriate interaction with the environment as circumstances change. We find that audition and vision implicitly interact, but certainly not in the way some neuropsychological tests of attention are organized. We live in a dynamically changing environment, and all of these networks eventually interact with the sensory and motor networks for adaptive functioning. Neuropsychological tests are not organized in these ways. Neuropsychological tests are often organized according to principles of face validity, and although this might represent logic based upon intuition, this way of organizing evaluation procedures certainly does not reflect the way brain-behavior relationships are organized within the brain. Untangling these network systems, or attempting to individually evaluate any single network, represents a significant challenge for neuropsychological assessment. In fact, the question remains whether or not a paradigm of this type can ever really be achieved. In any event, we firmly believe that certain modifications can be made within the way we administer current neuropsychological tests, and that certain evaluation procedures can be developed in order to assist in developing ways of measuring the functioning of these networks, and their interactions with subcortical systems.

References

1. Lezak, M. D., Howieson, D. B., Bigler, E. D., & Tranel, D. (2012). *Neuropsychological assessment* (5th ed.). New York, NY: Oxford University Press.
2. Koziol, L. F., & Budding, D. E. (2011). Pediatric neuropsychological testing: Theoretical models of test selection and interpretation. In A. Davis (Ed.), *Handbook of pediatric neuropsychology* (pp. 443–455). New York, NY: Springer.
3. Koziol, L. F., Budding, D. E., & Chidekel, D. (2013). *ADHD as a model of brain-behavior relationships*. New York, NY: Springer.
4. Koziol, L. F. (2014). *The myth of executive functioning: Missing elements in conceptualization, evaluation, and assessment*. New York, NY: Springer.
5. Keogh, B. K. (1994). A matrix of decision points in the measurement of learning disabilities (Chapter 2). In G. Reid Lyon (Ed.), *Frames of reference for the assessment of learning disabilities* (pp. 15–26). Baltimore, MD: Brookes Publishing.
6. Salmon, D. P., & Bondi, M. W. (2009). Neuropsychological assessment of dementia. *Annual Review of Psychology, 60*, 257–282.
7. Korkman, M., Kirk, U., Kemp, S., & Psychological Corporation. (2007). *NEPSY-II* (2nd ed.). San Antonio, TX: Harcourt Assessment.
8. Wechsler, D. (2014). *Wechsler intelligence scale for children* (5th ed.). San Antonio, TX: NCS Pearson.
9. Koziol, L. F., & Budding, D. E. (2009). *Subcortical structures and cognition: Implications for neuropsychological assessment*. New York, NY: Springer.
10. Cole, M. W., Bassett, D. S., Power, J. D., Braver, T. S., & Petersen, S. E. (2014). Intrinsic and task-evolved network architectures of the human brain. *Neuron, 83*(1), 238–251.
11. Cole, M. W., Reynolds, J. R., Power, J. D., Repovs, G., Anticevic, A., & Braver, T. S. (2013). Multi-task connectivity reveals flexible hubs for adaptive task control. *Nature Neuroscience, 16*(9), 1348–1355.
12. Freeman, J. B., & Ambady, N. (2011). A dynamic interactive theory of person construal. *Psychological Review, 118*(2), 247–279.
13. Freeman, J. B., & Ambady, N. (2011). Hand movements reveal the time-course of shape and pigmentation processing in face categorization. *Psychonomic Bulletin and Review, 18*(4), 705–712.
14. Martin, A. (2007). The representation of object concepts in the brain. *Annual Review of Psychology, 58*, 25–45.
15. Valyear, K. F., Chapman, C. S., Gallivan, J. P., Mark, R. S., & Culham, J. C. (2011). To use or to move: goal-set modulates priming when grasping real tools. *Experimental Brain Research, 212*(1), 125–142.
16. Hendriks-Jansen, H. (1996). *Catching ourselves in the act: situated activity, interactive emergence, evolution, and human thought* (Complex adaptive systems). Cambridge, MA: MIT Press.
17. Cisek, P., & Kalaska, J. F. (2010). Neural mechanisms for interacting with a world full of action choices. *Annual Review of Neuroscience, 33*, 269–298.
18. Koziol, L. F., Barker, L. A., & Jansons, L. (2015). Attention and other constructs: Evolution or revolution? *Applied Neuropsychology Child, 4*(2), 123–131.
19. Baron, I. S. (2004). *Neuropsychological evaluation of the child*. New York, NY: Oxford University Press.
20. Strauss, E., Sherman, E. M. S., Spreen, O., & Spreen, O. (2006). *A compendium of neuropsychological tests: Administration, norms, and commentary*. Oxford, England: Oxford University Press.
21. Ito, M. (1997). Cerebellar microcomplexes. In J. D. Schmahmann (Ed.), *The cerebellum and cognition* (pp. 475–489). San Diego, CA: Academic.
22. Goligher, J. C., & Hughes, E. S. R. (1951). Sensibility of the rectum and colon. Its role in the mechanism of anal continence. *Lancet, 1*, 543–547.
23. Lazarescu, A., Turnbull, G. K., & Vanner, S. (2009). Investigating and treating fecal incontinence: When and how. *Canadian Journal of Gastroenterology, 23*(4), 301–308.

24. Walker, H. K. (1990). Cranial nerve V: The trigeminal nerve (Chapter 61). In H. K. Walker, W. D. Hall, & J. W. Hurst (Eds.), *Clinical methods: The history, physical, and laboratory examinations* (3rd ed.). Boston, MA: Butterworths.
25. Dennis, R. E., Williams, W. W., Giangreco, M. F., & Cloninger, C. J. (1993). Quality of life as a context for planning and evaluation of services for people with disabilities: A review of the literature. *Exceptional Children, 59*, 499–512.
26. Moats, L. C. (1993). Spelling error interpretation: Beyond phonetic/dysphonetic dichotomy. *Annals of Dyslexia, 43*(1), 174–185.
27. Njiokiktjien, C. (2010). Developmental dyspraxias: Assessment and differential diagnosis. In D. Riva & C. Njiokiktjien (Eds.), *Brain lesion localization and developmental functions* (pp. 157–186). Montrouge, France: John Libbey Eurotext.
28. Welsh, M. C., & Pennington, B. F. (1988). Assessing frontal lobe functioning in children: Views from developmental psychology. *Developmental Neuropsychology, 4*(3), 199–230.
29. Koziol, L. F., & Lutz, J. T. (2013). From movement to thought: The development of executive function. *Applied Neuropsychology Child, 2*(2), 104–115.
30. Goldberg, E., Podell, K., Bilder, R., & Jaeger, J. (2000). *The executive control battery*. Sidney, New South Wales, Australia: Psych Press.
31. Denckla, M. B. (1985). Revised neurological examination for subtle signs. *Psychopharmacology Bulletin, 21*, 773–800.
32. Schacter, D. L., & Addis, D. R. (2007). The cognitive neuroscience of constructive memory: Remembering the past and imagining the future. *Philosophical Transactions of the Royal Society, B: Biological Sciences, 362*(1481), 773–786.
33. Mahon, B. Z., & Caramazza, A. (2009). Concepts and categories: A cognitive neuropsychological perspective. *Annual Review of Psychology, 60*, 27–51.
34. Asplund, C. L., Todd, J. J., Snyder, A. P., & Marois, R. (2010). A central role for the lateral prefrontal cortex in goal-directed and stimulus-driven attention. *Nature Neuroscience, 13*(4), 507–512.
35. Lewis, J. W., Beauchamp, M. S., & DeYoe, E. A. (2000). A comparison of visual and auditory motion processing in human cerebral cortex. *Cerebral Cortex, 10*(9), 873–888.

Chapter 3
The Normal Distribution of the Bell-Shaped Curve

"Progress is impossible without change, and those who cannot change their minds cannot change anything."

George Bernard Shaw

"Personally, I'm always ready to learn, although I do not always like being taught."

Winston Churchill

"In the middle of difficulty lies opportunity."

Albert Einstein

This chapter briefly reviews a few very basic statistical concepts that are necessary for interpreting neuropsychological tests. We discuss "why" and "how" these concepts underpin aspects of symptom identification, quantification, and diagnosis. Every clinician or student reading this chapter must have already come across these ideas and how to apply them. Nevertheless, sometimes we all take things for granted. Our approach towards evaluation might then turn mechanical; we can become too relaxed in our thinking when making test interpretations. Of course, this can lead towards increased false positive or false negative errors. A brief refresher never hurts. The diagnostician who is an advanced statistician can skip this review, and your decision to do so can be based upon reading the next few paragraphs. The student or examiner who is relatively new to the field and who is primarily focusing on clinical ideas should probably read the entire summary. However, most of this review focuses upon how statistics can be inadvertently misused in test interpretation. Perhaps for this reason, anyone who is uncertain about the ideas that are covered should consult the statistics book they used at some point in their education and/or training.

We all need to remember the obvious fact that the field of statistics did not develop to meet the needs of neuropsychology. Instead, neuropsychology relied upon the field of statistics so that certain needs inherent in the study of brain-behavior relationships

© Springer International Publishing Switzerland 2016
L.F. Koziol et al., *Large-Scale Brain Systems and Neuropsychological Testing*,
DOI 10.1007/978-3-319-28222-0_3

could be met. A few of neuropsychology's "needs" include quantification, determining differences in functioning between any particular patient and a reference group, and of course, experimental applications to name just a few areas. Neuropsychology "borrowed" certain ideas from statistics to serve the needs of its development. Statistics are basically guidelines applied to the testing and evaluation process which assist the neuropsychologist in structuring the process of test interpretation. Sometimes, the statistics we use can never represent a "perfect fit." For example, certain clinically important behaviors can never be identified or quantified through a statistical application. Attempts can be made to identify and quantify certain behaviors, but in our view, this represents a misapplication of statistics that only increases the likelihood of diagnostic error. For example, consider the "signs" of constructional dyspraxia, dyscalculia, stimulus-bound behavior, and disorientation to name less than a handful of behaviors that are symptoms we often identify. Applying a statistic to these observations results in a loss of the very meaning we should be attributing to the behavior. These are all very basic, simple examples of what we mean when we say meaningful neuropsychological evaluation can never be achieved by simply "going by the numbers." This viewpoint also emphasizes the distinction between "testing" and "evaluation."

The Normal Distribution

In certain diagnostic settings, there can be a need for quantification. For example, if an examiner believes in the construct of "general cognitive ability," the quantification provided by the intelligence quotient, or "IQ," immediately comes to mind. It is widely assumed and generally accepted that IQ follows what is termed a "normal distribution."

For the purpose of neuropsychological testing, whenever we think of a normal distribution, three statistical principles should immediately come to mind. First, a normal distribution always implies a bell-shaped curve. Second, if we actually drew this curve, the total area within this "curve" can immediately be concluded to equal a numeric value of 1. This is loosely another way of saying all cases fall somewhere within this area or curve. Third, and perhaps most importantly, the bell-shaped curve is symmetrical. If we drew a line down the middle of this curve, each half of this curve would be equal, representing 50 % of the area on each side. In statistics, the value assigned to each half of the area is 5. Figure 3.1 illustrates these statistical concepts. Therefore, if we accept the assumption that general intellectual ability is normally distributed, we are saying that the numeric values of an "IQ" test can be distributed within a bell-shaped curve, that all cases of "IQ" fall within the area of the curve and can be assigned a value of 1 (all cases = 1), and that all "IQ" scores are symmetrically distributed, with half of the cases falling on each side of the symmetrical curve. The exact middle of the curve can be understood as reflecting the mean or average level. Each number or value represents the exact same unit of quantification which further defines this "symmetry."

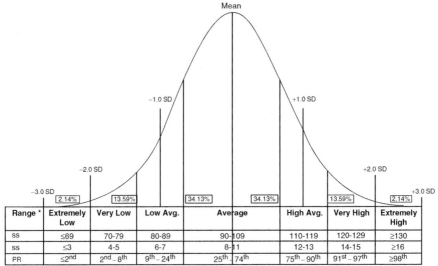

Fig. 3.1 The normal bell curve

In order to make these statistical concepts even more applicable to measurement for identifying differences, a "bell shaped curve" can be statistically refined by converting it into a "standard normal distribution," which includes two additional concepts. First, since our artificial line that divides the middle of the distribution is the statistical mean, statisticians convert this middle line, or "average," to a value of 0. Second, the "population standard" is an artificially derived term and it is automatically assigned a value of 1. This is also referred to as the "standard deviation." If we move 1 standard deviation in either direction, we illustrate where most of the "IQ" scores fall. Most IQ scores would be distributed within 1 standard deviation on either side of our middle, or average, line. From a statistical point of view, approximately 68 %, or the majority of the scores would fall between our first standard deviation above and below this average. By applying the appropriate statistical formula, we can further divide the bell shaped curve into distances 2 and 3 standard deviations above and below the mean—the "distances" from the mean score, with each statistical division representing a certain percentage of cases, specifically 95 and 98 % of cases, on either side of the average (as also illustrated in Fig. 3.1.) Any given "score" on an "IQ" test is converted to represent this statistical process, which then represents a "standard score," or how much that score deviates from the average range.

This methodology allows us to *categorize* each percentage of cases above and below the mean. For instance, within the first standard deviation band, where 68 % of the cases lie, we have the "average" range. A standard deviation above the mean becomes "high average," while a standard deviation below the mean becomes "low average." As we move 2 and 3 standard deviations above and below the mean, we construct the superior, very superior, borderline, and "deficient" ranges, depending upon where any particular test score lies above or below the average. Each categorization represents a smaller and smaller percentage of the cases as depicted within our original bell-shaped curve. In these ways, this methodology allows us to "quantify" any given person's test score, while simultaneously identifying the percentage of individual's who obtained a higher or lower score. We can even construct a "table" that lists the numeric values of our ranges that define each group we categorized.

A number of cognitive/behavioral functions appear to follow a normal distribution within the general population. We have seen how a normal distribution implies that there are gradients of characteristics being measured. Within this paradigm a portion of individuals in a given population will demonstrate accelerated or robust acquisition of a given function or ability, while others will manifest acceptable or average levels, and those remaining will demonstrate less ability or skill acquisition. The function being measured would theoretically follow a "bell shaped curve" which psychometrically would range from deficient or impaired to very superior. Importantly, when we apply this methodology, we are automatically accepting the assumption that the cognitive/behavioral function we are "testing" is normally distributed. This means we immediately accept the assumptions that the function/ cognitive skill/behavior follows the distribution of a bell shaped curve, that all individuals can be equally represented within this "curve," and that this distribution is symmetrical. Accepting these assumptions in interpreting test results can be problematic. For example, certain cognitions/behaviors, as cited above in our references to dyspraxia, disorientation, and stimulus-bound behavior, etc., simply do not follow a normal distribution within the general population. In other words, certain developmental processes and/or cases of loss of function do not follow this type of distribution, even though test scores can often be statistically derived in an attempt to measure these functions and behaviors. In reality, these types of functions likely follow a highly skewed distribution, while the interpretative meaning assigned to any deviation from the "skew" is pathological in each and every instance of occurrence. Although certain functions are skewed, most test publishers seem to prefer to transform these types of scores into a standard normal distribution, although the reasoning behind this transformation is unclear because it leads to errors in symptom identification and/or diagnosis.

Limitations of Standard Normal Distributions

In many instances, this type of distribution does not reveal much useful information. To illustrate the point, let's extend the concept of the bell shaped curve to its absurd logical conclusion. For example, if you were interested in purchasing certain types of clothing, such as sweatpants, the variable of interest would likely be waist size. Waist size can be measured in inches, or it can be represented within the construct of categorization. In this case, the variables of interest would change to waist size band, such as small, medium, large, or extra-large. This type of categorization has a very limited application. It does not tell us anything beyond one aspect of a clothing purchase. It would be very misleading to conclude that people came in four sizes, as in small, medium, large, and extra-large. A person might be very tall and with a small waist size; another individual might be very short and with a large waist size, etc. The variable of interest is limited and does not easily generalize to other variables. In converting to waist band size, we have generated a type of "composite quotient" that was then classified or categorized.

A similar example can be illustrated by knowing a person's IQ value. This type of measurement, which can be referred to as a "level of performance" criteria, says nothing about a person's cognitive assets, weaknesses, or deficits. It merely allows us to compare a person to some type of population sample. In developing a test of memory, we can similarly develop test scores, convert these scores into the properties of a bell-shaped curve, and then summarize the performances into borderline, low average, average, or high average "memory," etc. However, even though some people might have a "better" memory than others, is memory really normally distributed? Does memory really meet the characteristics and assumptions of a standard normal distribution? Does comparing a score on a memory test tell us anything about any given individual's IQ or does IQ tell us much about memory, even though the scores on the tests were converted into "standard scores" for statistically equivalent comparisons? Of course not! In fact, comparing all test scores to IQ scores, or "cognitive referencing," in not a recommended practice for interpretation [1]. This is closely related to our example of "waist band" telling us nothing about "height." So the assumptions we make when scoring tests and converting them into the proper statistical parameters for comparisons does not necessarily tell us anything we want to know; knowing about a person's global cognitive functioning says nothing about the probability of that same person having "good" memory. The variables of interest are completely different, despite the statistical equivalence of scores. And the categorization process is not at all informative; what exactly is "average" or "high average" memory? What is "borderline" range memory? These categorizations simply tell us nothing other than how one person compares to another, or to a group population, on any given test. With respect to "memory," a completely different comparison standard is required. One of the only relevant variables concerns how much information any given person acquired at "time 1," and then comparing that person's functioning to a delayed condition memory trial at "time 2." The variable of interest is remembering/forgetting, and this requires what is termed an individual comparison standard that has nothing to do with a group comparison standard. In an individual comparison standard, the individual in question literally acts as his or her own control, or point of reference. (This example was given only to illustrate the potential for misdiagnosis/symptom identification when certain statistical assumptions are made, and not to review all relevant variables of interest in examining anyone's "memory.") This type of measurement and categorization process becomes more ludicrous when we consider artificial constructs such as attention, executive functioning, and language. These "domains" are not unitary entities, these theoretical constructs have no universally agreed upon definitions within neuropsychology, and to scale and interpret these functions as if they followed a normalized standard distribution conveys no meaning at all about the functional construct in question. What exactly is "average" attention and/or executive functioning? We have seen these conclusions drawn in clinical practice, primarily when providing second opinion evaluations, while we admit that every practitioner, by definition, must be dealing with a skewed patient population or they would not present for evaluation to begin with. Therefore, other practitioners might not observe variability in test interpretation from other examiners. Scaling a person's test performance can be very useful as an anchor, or starting point. However, understanding the function being measured, and the statistical assumptions made and accepted, always need to be up-front in the examiner's mind, and not "taken for granted." Taking statistical processes for granted in interpreting tests is an examiner's source of error. Unfortunately, there are no formal standards of practice in clinical neuropsychology because this "error source" can easily be eliminated. We suggest that test publisher's include in the manual of every test the relevant information about whether or not the function being measured is normally distributed, and what statistical manipulations were performed in order to derive "scores" for that particular function.

Application and Misapplication of Statistical Processes

Determining the location of a function within the normal distribution has taken hold of the field of neuropsychology. We argue that this is the most common methodology for quantifying a variety of neurodevelopmental and neurocognitive processes. There is some utility and clinical relevance in quantifying the development of a particular function in relation to a patient's age-matched cohort. However, some functions are normally distributed while other functions are not, and this is where problems in test interpretation are often found.

Statistically speaking, the greater the number of skills, or even "items" required in completing a task to assess a particular function, the greater the likelihood that the function in question will follow the "normal" distribution [2]. For example, when someone performs within the "average" range of intelligence, this essentially means that after taking a behavioral sample, quantifying the behavior and statistically manipulating a variety of different neurocognitive functions in aggregate, the statistical outcome is equal to or better than at least 16 % of the individual's age-matched cohort. However, the process of transforming a behavior into a number, by running it through a variety of statistical operations, would seem to diminish the value of the original behavioral observation. Additionally, when aggregating a variety of neurocognitive processes that likely recruit a variety of neural systems, the value in the resulting number is diminished. In fact, an "average" performance on a given measure may in fact be highly misleading which may result in inaccurate assumptions and improper diagnoses. For instance, what does an average performance really tell us if the variables of interest lie within the individual, and not in comparison to any given group standard? What does the term "average" imply if it is based upon an aggregate of scores? In computing any average, there must be a high point and there must be a low point. If the variables of primary interest lie within this variability, then the process of computing an aggregate quotient actually masks exactly what we want to know.

Take for example an individual that obtains an "average" standard score on the Processing Speed Index of the Wechsler Scales. At face value the individual may be described as having average speed of thought or as being capable of completing basic neurocognitive tasks efficiently. There are many problems with this analysis in terms of what we know about neural system recruitment and in terms of the resulting interpretation. Relying on the use of a normative statistical process as the only way to analyze and interpret the data is a flawed approach. To further this very simple yet meaningful example, perhaps this same individual performed at the 25th percentile on the Coding subtest (ss = 8) while performing at the 75th percentile on the Symbol Search subtest (ss = 12). The aggregate statistical transformation results in an average PSI (SS = 100; 50th percentile). Suggesting this individual has average "processing speed" is inaccurate and may result in the clinician missing meaningful diagnostic information. Imaging studies [3] have demonstrated the Symbol Search and Coding subtests likely have different underlying neural substrates and, as such, putting them into a larger Index or "domain" is both misleading and neuroanatomically inaccurate. This same individual may demonstrate highly advanced "processing speed" on other Wechsler subtests which may be overlooked simply because the subtest is not included with the Processing Speed Index. If this individual earned numerous "bonus points" for speed on the Block Design subtest, this would indicate that the individual completed a constructional (novel problem-solving) task in a highly efficient manner, which we suggest would also constitute cognitive "processing speed". When standardized data is considered from this perspective, the practicing and aspiring neuropsychologist should begin to question the true clinical utility of transforming behaviors into standardized scores and domain analysis, the limitations inherent in this approach including masking the variables of interest, as well as the face validity of specific domain and score index names. The best "rule of thumb" to apply to test interpretation is to approach the matter with caution. To this end, we hope to advance the notion being championed by many in the field regarding the need for a paradigm shift in the field of neuropsychology. And at least one aspect of this "shift" is to ask reflective questions about what and how a function is being measured.

The utility of quantifying behavioral observations, running these raw scores through a variety of statistical operations and then quantifying one's performance along a normative distribution that presumably measures some sort of construct does not align with neuroanatomical findings [4]. Imaging studies have not resulted in the identification of compartmentalized "domains" such as processing speed, attention, working memory, etc. Forcing behaviors into artificially defined constructs or domains is inconsistent with contemporary findings within the neurosciences and, as such, is a relatively limited methodology for interpretation. Consider the commonly tested and reported general ability (IQ) composite standard score as we described it above. What does this score tell us about the individual in terms of neuropsychological functioning? Ultimately what is the clinical utility of a single

IQ standard score? IQ is arguably an outdated, a-theoretical concept that has been relatively unchanged since it was initially conceptualized many years ago [5]. Even though IQ tests were never intended to be applied as neuropsychological tools, IQ tests are routinely used in neuropsychological testing. Despite dramatic changes in the field of neuroscience, neuropsychology has held and, in many ways, supported the idea of an IQ. There is no way to obtain a single number to quantify the functioning of the numerous integrated and interactive neuropsychological systems in the brain. Experimental investigations that inform us about brain-behavior relationships do not include IQ tests as a form of measurement of cognitive functions. In fact, in many cases the IQ score is misleading and, as a result, may in fact be harmful to our patients. Clinical neuropsychological evaluation should focus on the integrity of various neuropsychological "systems" with respect to how they operate in isolation and in integration, whenever the variables of interest are identified and known. When using a systems approach to test interpretation and evaluation, a methodology that aligns with what is known about understanding the functioning of brain networks (e.g., frontal-parietal network, dorsal attention network, ventral attention network, etc.) will be of greater clinical value than the use of a single number to quantify the patient's IQ or a patient's functioning within an arbitrary and a-theoretical construct or "domain." We further discuss a systems approach to neuropsychological assessment in future sections of this text. We also argue that many tests currently in use do not easily align with what is known about large scale brain networks, and that this calls for alterations in the way we administer tests. This also speaks to the need for the development of new tests and methodologies.

Chance Variation and Statistical Versus Clinical Significance

There are inherent dangers in an over-reliance on standardized scores as the primary methodology in test interpretation. To provide additional practical evidence, consider a case in which an individual functions within the superior or very superior range on the Verbal Comprehension Index, but functions within the high average range on the Perceptual Reasoning Index. From a statistical point of view, this type of discrepancy is significant; however, dependent upon other factors that we might know about the given individual, that type of variability might not reflect any clinical significance whatsoever. This is based upon a simple statistical principle. To begin with, the entire set of Wechsler scales, as well as many other measures of intellectual functioning, is based upon the idea that everyone within the general population is good at performing certain tasks and not so good at performing other tasks (i.e., the individual shows a pattern of strengths and weaknesses). When an individual performs extremely well in one area, in this case the verbal domain, the likelihood that the Perceptual Reasoning Index score in our example falls significantly below the Verbal Comprehension Index score can simply occur by statistical chance, having little to do with the given individual's cognitive-adaptive capability structure. This would represent a false positive finding if statistical significance was considered to equal clinical significance. On the other hand, if an individual had a documented lesion, by assumption within the right cerebral hemisphere, this type of difference might be clinically significant, although this score might continue to fall within the high average range on the Perceptual Reasoning Index, when compared to a normative group standard. In this case, a finding that was statistically significant is also clinically significant, and interpreting the score as a matter of chance variation would represent a false negative finding.

The exact same interpretation would be true if an individual had a Perceptual Reasoning Index score that fell within the superior to very superior range, with a Verbal Comprehension Index score that fell, perhaps, within the low average to average range. Simply because the individual performed well on Perceptual Reasoning Index subtests, and earned lower scores on Verbal Comprehension Index subtests, this type of finding might be a manifestation of statistical chance variability. In this case, an interpretation of clinical significance derived from statistical significance would, indeed, represent a false positive finding.

Conversely, although the individual might function at a seemingly respectable level on the Verbal Comprehension Index and well on the Perceptual Reasoning Index in comparison to same-age peers, the reason for this lack of statistically significant difference might mask the presence of a documented brain lesion, or perhaps a developmental language disorder. In this case, minimizing perhaps a minor difference between these two Index scores would represent a false negative finding. Similarly, when an individual has verbal scores within a low average and sometimes borderline statistical range, the greater the likelihood that the so-called performance scores are notably higher generally increases as a matter of chance variation alone [6]. As described in the previous chapter, a level of performance criteria does not explain the reason for that performance. Similarly, statistical significance does not equate to clinical significance.

These theoretical examples represent simple, yet exemplary samples of the types of misrepresentations or misinterpretations that can be made when interpreting test performances according to a quantified level of performance criteria alone, while assuming that the functions in question all follow the normal distribution of a bell-shaped curve. Therefore, once again, we reiterate there are interpretive, diagnostic, and clinical limitations when considering a level of performance criteria while assuming that the skill sets in question always follow a standard normal distribution. Cognitive development, deterioration, decline, or impairment can never be determined simply on the basis of a level of performance criteria (i.e., scores). Similarly, comparing every cognitive skill to IQ, a practice known as "cognitive referencing," will very frequently result in misinterpretation when skill sets are assumed to follow a normal distribution but in fact, they do not.

Similarly, a statistically significant difference between sets of scores, or even a lack thereof, has nothing to do with the level of possible severity of impairment. The categorizations of low-average, average, superior, etc., cannot be applied to predicting whether or not any given individual is significantly impaired in any given function. As just one example, level of impairment cannot even be inferred when the appropriate individual comparison standard is applied in the interpretation of memory tests. An extremely capable individual can easily achieve scores within the "average" range on every index of a memory test if that person had "superior" memory premorbidly. And even though "average" scores were obtained, that individual might be so impaired that they can no longer adequately function in the practical occupational setting. The point that neuropsychological tests have limited ecological validity is often overlooked, and a false negative finding in cases of this type are misleading and can be harmful to the patient [7].

More About Statistical Conversions Versus Normal Distributions

The reader may question what some of the problems are that are inherent in transforming test performances into a bell-shaped curve. There are many neuro-cognitive behaviors/skills that should be considered "have" or "have-not" neu-rocognitive behaviors/skills. These behaviors/skills do not follow a normal distribution. Instead, dichotomous distributions are inherent in numerous behaviors. As just one primary example, phonological processing has nothing to do with a bell-shaped curve. Forcing phonological processing into a normal distribution actually violates the concept, as deficits in phonological processing are pathognomonic of neurocognitive impairment [8]. In fact, scores on measures of phonological processing that fall below the 50th percentile represent deficits in acquisition and are predictive of reading, writing, and language disorders [9]. Ninety percent of the population with deficits in phonological awareness/pro-cessing experience difficulties in learning to read [9] and, as such, this is a critical function to accurately measure.

Phonological processing can be evaluated in a variety of ways. For instance, in 4 year old children, phonological awareness and phonological processing often may be measured by having a child tap out the number of different sounds within a word, rhyme words, or identify similar phonemes and morphemes. At this age, phonological processing is very difficult to measure, as many 4 year olds have difficulties with these phonological processing tasks. By forcing these behaviors/skill into a normative distribution we increase the possibility of false negatives and miss opportunities to intervene during critical windows of neurodevelopment. It is well accepted within the psychological and commercial testing industries that the earlier a child is tested the less test-retest reliability [10, 11]. By the age of 5 years, nearly 1 year later, approximately 50 % of children are capable of tapping out the number of different sounds within a word, rhyming effectively, and identifying the location of phonemes and morphemes within words [12]. Half of the 5 year old children are capable of performing a task that almost none of the 4 year old children were able to perform. By the time a child reaches 7 years of age, 90 % are capable of demonstrating behaviors/skills that are presumed to underlie phonological awareness and phonological processing [12]. The point we are making is that a skill such as phonological processing does not follow the normal distribution of the bell-shaped curve. Instead the skill follows a highly skewed distribution. It represents a pathognomonic or specific sign in terms of its predictive value. Transforming this type of performance into a normal distribution violates the purpose of the cognitive skill and its predictive interpretation.

To use an example, assume for a moment that visual acuity follows a normal "bell-shaped" distribution curve. If a child's visual acuity was consistent with or better than 37 % of his or her age-matched cohort, many parents might elect to intervene or correct the child's visual deficits. Yet, psychometrically speaking, the 37th percentile falls comfortably within the average range (16–84th percentile). Despite falling within the average range on the bell-shaped curve, the child's vision being consistent with only 37 % of their age-matched cohort would likely warrant corrective lenses. To take our example a step further, if a child's vision were at the 25th percentile, being equal to or worse than 75 % of the child's age-matched peers, this would be considered a significant visual deficit with correction being strongly indicated. Yet, in a "normal" distribution, the 25th percentile again falls comfortably within the average range (16–84th percentile) when using a statistically methodology to quantify performance. Vision which warrants correction, despite being within the average range, would not be considered to be "intact," yet when using a normative distribution to analyze neuropsychological measures, the term "average" is synonymous with "intact." This is misleading and, in fact, represents a false negative interpretation.

The point we are making is that many neurocognitive processes do not follow a normally distributed pattern, and the identification of pathognomonic signs may be a more salient methodology in terms of interpretation, diagnosis, and intervention. In the case of phonological processing, a 5 year old child that performs at the 25th percentile is, in fact, demonstrating delays in phonological development regardless of the fact that the child's score falls within the average range on the standard bell-curve. Children who score at or below the level of the 25th percentile within a normative population on measures of phonological development and phonological processing are significantly more likely to demonstrate reading, writing, and language delays when compared to age-mates who demonstrate "intact" phonological processing (i.e., scores equal to or better than 50 % of the normative sample) [9]. Therefore, as is the case with vision, although the child's score may be within the "average" range, intervention is indicated in such cases to support phonological development and to reduce the likelihood of the child developing additional disorders (i.e., reading, writing, language, etc.). Underdevelopment of phonological processing is pathognomonic in nature.

To provide another example, consider the feeding abilities of a neonate, including the ability to latch and suck. The neonate's ability to latch, suck, and feed is indicative of his or her overall neuromotor development and, as such, is predictive of future neurodevelopmental delays. Metrics could be developed, constructed and used to quantify the neonate's feeding abilities (e.g., suck strength, rate, extraction volume, etc.); however, such metric information would be arbitrary and would provide little information beyond a particular neonate's performance relative to that of other neonates. Presently, what is known is that difficulties in feeding predict future neurodevelopmental delays and, as such, represent pathognomonic signs [13].

Walking is another neurodevelopmental skill that does not follow a normative distribution. There could be ways of quantifying a child's walking proficiency, such as assessing walking speed, the ratio of falling in relation to steps taken, the time it takes a child to move from one location to another, gait pattern, etc. Using various metrics, it would be possible to place a child's walking ability into a normative distribution; however, one must question the utility of doing so. It is known that by that age of 12 months children should be walking independently. When they are not, it is a sign of concern about the child's neurodevelopment. The use of a normative distribution is arbitrary, irrelevant, and of no clinical utility. Either the child is able to walk independently at 12 months, or the child is not.

The use of an arbitrary statistical threshold for determining what is "pathological" and what is "normal" may be harmful to our patients. When using the bell-shaped curve to analyze and interpret data, we are doomed to numerous false negatives and, as a result, we miss critical opportunities to support our patients' neurodevelopment. Ultimately, the goal of neuropsychological assessment is to identify pathology so that interventions may be developed and implemented to enhance one's brain-behavior functioning. To this end we hope those in our field may reconsider the utility of our current psychometric approach to test interpretation and analysis. Quantification has its place, but not all functions of clinical utility can be captured by a number. Two quotations immediately come to mind. For example, Seneca once stated, *"It is the quality rather than the quantity that matters,"* and Albert Einstein stated, *"Not everything that can be counted counts, and not everything that counts can be counted."* We hope these quotes will cause some readers to pause, stop, and think about the complexities of the neurobiologic substrates of behaviors, and the methodologies we employ to measure them.

References

1. Fletcher, J. M., & Dennis, M. (2010). Spina bifida and hydrocephalus. In K. O. Yeates, M. D. Ris, & H. G. Taylor (Eds.), *Pediatric neuropsychology: Research, theory, and practice* (2nd ed., pp. 3–25). New York, NY: Guilford.
2. Grinstead, C. M., & Snell, J. L. (2012). *Introduction to probability*. Providence, RI: American Mathematical Society.
3. Sweet, L. H., Paskavitz, J. F., O'Connor, M. J., Browndyke, J. N., Wellen, J. W., & Cohen, R. A. (2005). FMRI correlates of the WAIS-III Symbol Search subtest. *Journal of the International Neuropsychological Society, 11*, 471–476.
4. Insel, T. R. (2014). The NIMH research domain criteria (RDoC) project: Precision medicine for psychiatry. *American Journal of Psychiatry, 171*(4), 395–397.
5. Sparrow, S. S., & Davis, S. M. (2000). Recent advances in the assessment of intelligence and cognition. *Journal of Child Psychology and Psychiatry, and Allied Disciplines, 41*(1), 117–131.
6. Walsh, K. W. (1978). *Neuropsychology: A clinical approach*. Oxford, England: Churchill Livingstone.
7. Chaytor, N., & Schmitter-Edgecombe, M. (2003). The ecological validity of neuropsychological tests: A review of the literature on everyday cognitive skills. *Neuropsychology Review, 13*(4), 181–197.
8. Habib, M. (2000). The neurological basis of developmental dyslexia. *Brain, 123*(12), 2373–2399.
9. Hogan, T. P., Catts, H. W., & Little, T. D. (2005). The relationship between phonological awareness and reading: Implications for the assessment of phonological awareness. *Language, Speech, and Hearing Services in Schools, 36*(4), 285–293.

10. Sattler, J. M. (2008). *Assessment of children* (5th ed.). San Diego, CA: Jerome M. Sattler.
11. Strauss, E., Sherman, E. M. S., & Spreen, O. (2006). *A compendium of neuropsychological tests: Administration, norms, and commentary.* Oxford, England: Oxford University Press.
12. Bishop, D. V. M., Nation, K., & Patterson, K. (2014). When words fail us: Insights into language processing from developmental and acquired disorders. *Philosophical Transactions of the Royal Society, B: Biological Sciences, 369*(1634), 20120403. http://doi.org/10.1098/rstb.2012.0403.
13. National Health and Medical Research Council. (2012). *Infant feeding guidelines.* Canberra, ACT, Australia: National Health and Medical Research Council.

Chapter 4
Beyond the Bell-Shaped Curve

"Failure is only the opportunity to begin again more intelligently."

Henry Ford

"Excellence is to do a common thing in an uncommon way."

Booker T. Washington

Intra-individual and Other Test Score Comparisons

The prior chapter demonstrated that referring only to a level of performance criteria tells us little, if anything, about any given person's clinical status. Assuming all cognitive functions can be understood within the symmetry of a statistical standard normal distribution runs a notably increased risk of making interpretive errors. Tests designed to assess the integrity of medial temporal lobe system functions provide a salient example of this issue. An assessment of anterograde amnesia, defined as the inability to learn new factual, semantic information, immediately comes to mind. When attempting to assess an individual's ability to learn and retain, comparison to an external normative group standard might even become totally irrelevant. Certain inferential conclusions can be diagnostically misleading. Consider the following test score data from the California Verbal Learning Test, 2nd Edition (CVLT II):

Test results		
		Age-corrected
CVLT-II	Raw	z-Score
List A		
Trial 1	6	−1.0
Trial 2	7	
Trial 3	7	

© Springer International Publishing Switzerland 2016
L.F. Koziol et al., *Large-Scale Brain Systems and Neuropsychological Testing*,
DOI 10.1007/978-3-319-28222-0_4

Test results		
		Age-corrected
CVLT-II	Raw	z-Score
Trial 4	9	
Trial 5	10	−4.0
List B	6	−1.0
Short delay free recall	9	−2.0
Long delay free recall	10	−2.0
Recognition	13 of 16	−4.0

These data allow us to illustrate four critically important points. First, comparing any given person's level of performance to a group norm is of very limited use in the evaluation of the learning and memory functions that are governed by the medial temporal lobe memory system. Second, this example allows us to describe the functions and processes relevant to this system. Third, it provides the opportunity for us to demonstrate how the methodology of test interpretation is directly derived from the neuro-anatomic substrates of that system. Fourth, it allows us to introduce a systematic way for interpreting memory tests while introducing the methodology of the *individual comparison standard*, or *relevant test score comparisons,* when the subject serves as his/her own control standard. In fact, a word list learning test that is well constructed is the only task that instantly comes to mind that illustrates level of performance, pattern analysis through test score comparisons, and pathognomonic signs, in aggregate, simultaneously for appropriate test interpretation—three separate methods of inference are applied for interpreting the data.

When approaching this particular set of test results, the examiner should immediately be struck by the idea that *statistics can easily tell us a lie.* For example, the z-scores are telling us that after hearing the exact same material for five consecutive trials, this person has a "negative" learning slope, because the individual performed at a level of only one standard deviation below the mean on the first trial, but four standard deviations below the mean after the fifth trial! But are these test data really pointing to that conclusion? Of course not!

The patient's "raw score" numbers clearly demonstrate a positive learning slope. The patient retrieved 6, 7, 7, 9, and 10 words across the five consecutive trails. So "learning," as defined by the person's voluntary or free recall, presumably reveals the acquisition of 10 words after starting out with an immediate recall trial of retrieving 6 words. However, when comparing this subject's performance to the age-appropriate group norm, he/she did not retrieve nearly as much information as their age-matched cohorts. *And, across all five consecutive trials, this is all the statistical norms are telling us. It is actually more important to interpret these "raw scores" without the group comparison, particularly if the issue is assessing the acquisition of information. Without this raw score information, the interpreter of these results is handicapped.* We cannot use the statistical conversion z-scores to tell us if this person is acquiring information as indexed by voluntary retrieval/recall. We seldom need these z-scores unless we are in the rare situation when what needs to be known is the group comparison. However, the z-scores do provide the examiner with sort of an anchor point as to how quickly this person *learns and retrieves newly presented information independently, on his or her own.* Nevertheless, the neophyte examiner might be "tricked" by inferring that this person actually "forgot" or was unable to retrieve as much information on trial 5 as they did on trial 1. And this illustration is not at all dramatic. This pattern of "raw" and z-scores occurs on a reasonably frequent basis. So three interpretive points emerge from this example. First, group comparison data are clearly not always the interpretive methodology of choice. Second, there is nothing the matter with using the "raw score" data, a summary of the patient's actual product. Third, the appropriate interpretive methodology here is the individual comparison standard—by comparing trial 1 with trial 5, the patient served the purpose of acting as his/her own control. And this was the *only way* we were able to determine that this person was learning information as referenced by free or voluntary retrieval.

The Medial Temporal Lobe Memory System

In order to interpret and assess the integrity of the medial temporal lobe memory system, we believe it is essential to understand its neuro-biologic substrate. This understanding literally provides the anchor point for test interpretation because the neuro-anatomic underpinnings of this system inform us about "what" is going on during test administration, and often times "why" this is occurring. A complete review of this system is beyond the limited scope of this chapter, but we can provide all the basic concepts that are necessary for evaluating this system. Knowing these concepts will provide a firm foundation for understanding how and why this system is or is not affected in various disease processes, enabling the reader to navigate through the literature about the functioning of this system in both health and disease. Any reader who is not conversant in the neuro-anatomy of this system should review Squire [1] and Eichenbaum [2]. This information is foundational for interpreting the remainder of our example. We are attempting to practice what we preach, that knowing about brain systems and knowing about the characteristics of tests are critical to test interpretation and evaluation.

Anterograde amnesia has four characteristics [3]. These features can be summarized as follows:

1. The subject is unable to retain newly presented information
2. The amnesia is global; this means the amnesia affects every sensory modality;
3. Immediate recall is intact;
4. General intellectual functioning, usually as measured by one of the WIS tests, is intact.

The medial temporal lobe memory system is "old" from a phylogenetic point of view [4]. In addition, this is a *recognition memory system.* Its original adaptive purpose had nothing to do with the voluntary or free, verbal recall of information. Humans have access to this system both through active verbal expression and recognition, but it remains a recognition system. As such, the most sensitive index of the integrity of this system, which evolved for the adaptive advantage of the retention of sensory experiences, is evaluated through the recognition trial of a word list learning test, such as the tests in the CVLT series [5]. Design recall tasks, sometimes called "non-verbal" learning/memory tests, are much more often than not confounded by the component of drawing. We can only retain what we originally attended to, so design recall tasks which might include a recognition trial are potentially flawed; unless the subject initially "paid attention" to design recall elements as presented in recognition trials, a lack of retention might not be the issue at hand at all. This is a subtle point that can lead an examiner towards false positive interpretive error. When trying to assess retention without active verbal expression, a *well constructed* facial learning and memory test represents a superior choice. In any case, regardless of modality of administration, learning and memory tasks designed to assess the medial temporal lobe memory system recruit *bilateral* activation of both cerebral hemispheres [6]. In any event, the reader would be correct in assuming that the medial temporal lobe memory system allows sensory experiences to persist, or to be retained. Therefore, in a systematic learning and memory examination, the first step is to assess the recognition component of the test. *Assessing this learning and memory system through active verbal expression or through drawing are unnecessary and in certain cases can be misleading. These variables remain important because they assess retrieval functions.* In any event, in our example, we immediately know there is no anterograde amnesia. The individual was able to retrieve 10 words on the 5th trial, and recognize 13 words in the recognition paradigm. So this "raw score" *comparison* immediately tells us more information was retained than the person could demonstrate on free recall trails, which is the next step in systematic memory test interpretation. (Nearly everyone is able to identify more information than they can actively retrieve.) However, we can conclude there is no memory disturbance.

Trials 1 through 5 are a rough index of how much information was acquired (measured by free recall) as well as providing at least some data about how quickly that information was learned. There is no evidence of inconsistent retrieval. The learning slope is shallow. There were no intrusions and no perseverations. Therefore, in this brief analysis, we can safely conclude that immediate recall is a bit limited but intact, that this individual learns factual information more slowly than expected, but whatever information this person learned was retained, although he/she did not learn as much information as their peer group. And given these limited data, these remain important conclusions, particularly if the referral question focused on neuropsychological memory disturbance since there is no anterograde amnesia. Importantly, the assumed diagnostic question of this case can be answered by simply reviewing the "raw score" data. The "normal distribution" is irrelevant, peer group comparisons are peripheral to the diagnostic question, and the most significant interpretations are derived from an individual comparison standard; the person served as his/her own control, with conclusions emerging from comparing one relevant aspect of the test performance with another.

Just because recognition paradigms are important to assessing the MTL system does not mean that people do not have access to the content of the information within it. The MTL remains an important "hub" region of the DMN. This was described in *ADHD as a Model of Brain-Behavior Relationships* [19] and *The Myth of Executive Functioning* [20]. The content of this system is relied upon for "EF" and decision-making, which was the *The Myth of Executive Functioning* [20]. However, using this information is one issue; trying to measure retention is quite another matter. The content of memory can often be relied upon *implicitly*. (Please review with the previously mentioned volumes if this distinction is unclear.)

The same individual comparison standard is applicable to a pathological case of memory disorder. Consider the following distribution of scores on the CVLT from a 63 years old male:

Test results		
		Age-corrected
CVLT	Raw	z-Score
List A		
Trial 1	7	0
Trial 2	8	
Trial 3	10	
Trial 4	12	
Trial 5	14	1.0
List B	6	0
Short delay free recall	10	0
Long delay free recall	9	0
Recognition	9 of 16	−3.0
False positives	9	+3.0
Free recall intrusions	8	+2.0

In this particular case, aspects of the z-score profile appear to be contradictory, but only when these scores are interpreted without making the appropriate intra-individual score comparisons and without *integrating* this data set. A group norm comparison is clearly misleading. If the recognition anchor point is "missed," the Long Delay Free Recall condition as described by a z-score is within the "average" range. However, recognition memory, perhaps the single best indicator of information retention, is 3 standard deviations below the mean. In addition, the next relevant dimension of the recognition paradigm, the number of "False Positive" errors, is also 3 standard deviations different even from normal control subjects. Therefore, recognition recall, one of our most important features of a memory evaluation, is contaminated by the patient's memory confusion; memory is therefore unreliable. But this conclusion can easily be inferred by the "raw scores" alone if one possesses an appropriate understanding of the MTL system as primarily serving an *accurate* information retention function. It is also notable that after five consecutive trials, Free Recall was "high average" (to reiterate, we believe this is an inappropriate neuropsychological classification nomenclature), and again, Long Delay Free Recall is at the "average" group comparison level. So what is the matter with possessing "average" memory?

The "raw score" data clearly demonstrate an inability to retrieve, or perhaps more appropriately in this case, "remember," 5 words after about 20 min. This is approximately a third of the information the person was initially capable of retrieving on trial 5. Similarly, on Free Recall trials, there were a significant number of retrieval errors or "intrusions." Therefore, when implementing the *individual comparison standard,* with the patient acting as his own control or point of reference, there is no question about these data representing memory disorder. In fact, this is the type of profile obtained from a patient with Alzheimer's disease. The data pattern is entirely consistent with a deterioration in semantic networks [7]. However, when making a normative group comparisons alone, the z-score pattern looks confusing. So in order to interpret these data properly, the interpreter needs to know about the MTL system, the disease pattern of Alzheimer's disease (a discussion of AD is well beyond the scope of our illustrative example), the way in which statistics can be used in neuropsychology, as well as a comprehensive understanding of the inferential methodology of the individual comparison standard. What is remarkable about both case samples is that all the relevant conclusions can be inferred without making reference to any other tests that were administered; this is the power available to the examiner who understands neuro-anatomical substrates of tests and how to interpret these "tools" systematically.

The following case of a 27 years old woman with approximately 16 years of education is initially even more confusing, particularly for the neophyte examiner in training, or the neuropsychologist first entering the field of clinical practice. This individual complains of difficulties with word finding, forgetfulness, problems with "remembering to remember," with a historic diagnosis of ADHD and symptoms of depression; the patient was assessed under the influence of her medication prescription with the chronic administration of Concerta and Wellbutrin:

Wechsler Memory Scale, 4th Edition (WMS-IV)

Subtest	Raw score	Scaled score	Percentile
Logical memory I	23	9	37
Logical memory II	24	10	50
Logical memory recognition	23	–	26–50 %

Rey Complex Figure Test and Recognition Trial (RCFT)

Subtest	Raw score	T score	Percentile
Copy	33	–	6–10

Subtest	Raw score	T score	Percentile
Immediate recall	20	41	18
Delayed recall	19.5	39	14
Recognition	22	53	62

California Verbal Learning Test, 2nd Edition (CVLT-II)

Subtest	Raw score	Standard score
Trial 1	7	−0.5
Trial2	9	−0.5
Trial 3	11	−0.5
Trial 4	13	0
Trial 5	13	−0.5
Trials 1–5 total	53	48 (T score)
Trial B	7	0
Short delay free recall	10	−0.5
Short delay cued recall	8	−2
Long delay free recall	10	−1
Long delay cued recall	7	−2.5
Semantic clustering	0.5	−0.5
Total repetitions	6	0
Total intrusions	4	0.5
Total hits	11	−4
Total false positives	1	0
Forced choice recognition % total accuracy	100	

Intrusions: elephant, shelf,

False Positives: elephant

To begin with, the narrative recall of the *Weschler Memory Scale—Fourth Edition* [8] do not suggest anterograde amnesia in any way at all. None of the score comparisons on that subtest imply any impairment whatsoever. It remains notable that the woman's "raw score points" generate such seemingly large statistical differences when in fact, the "raw score" data are essentially equivalent. And every examiner always needs to keep in mind that *narrative recall tasks are typically thematic. These are structured, organized tasks that can actually assist in the initial encoding of information and it's retention because it allows the person to rely upon the natural organization of language. In addition, verbatim recall is not required as it is on word list learning tasks. These factors can, and do influence "learning and memory" as demonstrated by the free, voluntary memory indices. These factors are exactly what is missing from word list learning and memory tasks and in many instances represent the reasoning behind administering both types of subtests.*

At first glance, the "total hits," or more accurately the recognition scores look problematic, regardless of "numeric" choice of interpretive index. With a "raw score" index of 11, compared to a Trial 5 production of 13, and Short and Long recall productions of 8 and 10 words respectively, inconsistent information retrieval is implied at the minimum, while the recognition recall trial actually implies information forgetting—a lack of information storage or retention. It can also be argued that the performances in "cued" conditions support these conclusions. However, there is a subtle clue in these data that do not support a diagnostic conclusion of a disorder of the medial temporal memory system. And that clue clearly emerges in the person's 100 % correct performance on the forced choice, yes-no recognition that requires the subject to indicate whether a long list of stimulus words read to them were on any list at all. And now the data very quickly become neuro-anatomically consistent.

This person's data are telling us that her medial temporal lobe system which functions for the purpose of the retention of newly presented information is intact. This is evident from the WMS-IV Logical Memory subtest and from the yes-no identification/recognition trial. She is also telling us that she learns and retains thematic information, which often mimics conversational discourse, without any more or less difficulty than anyone else her age within the standardization population for that narrative recall subtest. However, she is also "saying" that when she is left to rely upon her own organizational resources to acquire and accurately recall new information, she has significant trouble in recollecting the temporal ordering of information according to the time sequence of when the information [9]. She is uncertain if the data she heard were presented on List A or List B. Here is where the "confusion" lies within this data pattern, initially suggested by the contrast between the "total hits" score and the entirely accurate "yes-no" recognition score; this conclusion, consistent with the neuroanatomical substrate of the test, is further supported by the intrusion and perseveration "scores." Although not statistically significant, the performances can be explained by the same "anterior brain system" implications [10]. Finally, inconsistencies are evident in her self-retrieval of information.

And the Rey Complex Figure Test [11] can easily be integrated with similar conclusions. Her initial copying of the figure "missed" three elements (out of a total of 36), generating the skewed distribution of performance of this task. All of the "forgetting" occurred within 3 min of initially drawing the figure—the 3 min "immediate recall" trial is actually an incidental recall trial. If an examiner closely reviews the normative standards of the task, almost any "normal control" subject with a perfect copy score of 36 raw score points can "forget" a seemingly significant amount of information and continue to perform within an "average range" after 3 min. With this in mind, the "raw score" profile is equivalent when comparing incidental recall, delayed recall, and recognition recall, making it extremely difficult, if not impossible, to argue an impairment in medial temporal lobe learning and memory system (please refer to the test manual for test score comparisons). However, taking all these data together, in aggregate, there is considerable support for her complaints of forgetfulness, word retrieval difficulties, in addition to the organizational difficulties inferred from this test profile. Furthermore, the initially appearing "inconsistent" data become quite cohesive, coherent, and consistent in pointing to involvement of frontal-striatal systems, in contrast to primary medial temporal lobe memory formation deficits [12]. Additionally, there is some suggestion in the literature that medications such as Wellbutrin can contribute to the subjective experience of word-finding deficits (Personal communication—Jonathon C. Gamze, MD, 2011). However, whether or not aspects of her learning and memory profile might be associated with the iatrogenic effects of treatment cannot be etiologically determined.

Interim Conclusions

We have discussed how certain cognitive functions cannot be referenced according to the assumptions inherent in accepting the normal standard distribution. We have demonstrated this through a "blind analysis" of data that can be gathered by anyone in clinical practice. Individual test score comparisons were illustrated as an appropriate methodology for learning and memory tasks. Our examples illustrated how and why a knowledge of brain systems, tests and how they are constructed, are all critical to clinical interpretation. Although our analyses were intentionally not exhaustive, we reviewed how this level of knowledge can be applied towards making powerful inferences and diagnostic conclusions, even with data that at first might seem limited and even contradictory.

More About Test Pattern Analysis

The "level of performance" methodology, because of its inherent limitations, can only be an initial step for test interpretation. However, individual comparison standards and pattern analysis lie at the heart of substantive, efficient, and accurate neuropsychological test interpretation. Unfortunately, these are the most difficult levels of inference to understand. A knowledge of functional neuroanatomy is a very strong underpinning for the neuropsychologist to rely upon because this guides the examiner in knowing which data comparisons to make and which ones should be avoided. The set of test data being interpreted *always need to make anatomical sense.* And functional neuroanatomy can always be learned and updated by staying current with the literature. These days, it is incumbent upon the practitioner to understand large scale brain networks and systems. An understanding of what a test purports to measure, how the test was constructed, and the neuro-biologic substrates of that test are equally important factors. However, test manuals often provide little information in this regard, while many times a test is based upon an author's/publisher's idiosyncratic definition of any given function that might be in question. Some tests are even a-theoretical [13]. So considerable knowledge and experience are required in order to make sense of pattern analysis. This leads to synergistic test interpretation as our previous learning and memory examples have demonstrated— the test score comparisons tell us something brand new, information about a person's functioning that would never be inferred when interpreting a test, or aspects of a test, in isolation. Unfortunately, the opposite is also true; gaps within a clinician's knowledge base generates variability in the practitioner's work product, and sometimes the extent of this variability is unacceptable because it compromises the conclusions of the work product.

While a typical neuropsychological evaluation consists of numerous tests and subtests, the examiner must understand what these various tests might have in common and how they might differ, even if only in subtle ways. Without knowing what cognitive processes are necessary for successful task completion, it is impossible to determine what any task measures, and how performance on that task might relate to another task that has been administered. The clinical neuropsychologist must have an understanding of even subtle test attributes, and must thoughtfully analyze why an individual patient might perform poorly on one task but not on another when both tasks would presumably fall under the same domain of functioning or presumably measure the same, if not similar, cognitive processes. When a clinician is armed with this knowledge, pattern analysis or test score comparisons become synergistic with respect to interpretive value. Furthermore, this global knowledge base needs to be derived from empirical fact, and not clinical intuition. For example, the Tower of London test and the Tower of Hanoi tests are both considered tests of planning and organization; however, in interpretive reality, these tests simply do not correlate highly with one another in clinical populations. Therefore, these are two different tasks that do not evaluate the exact same neurocognitive functions, even though intuition and face validity might indicate otherwise (To explore this matter further, the interested reader is referred to *Subcortical Structures and Cognition*, 2009, Springer Publications [14].

For example, the Wisconsin Card Sorting Test (WCST) is considered a rule-based category learning test. The examinee is required to sort cards into three different categories, specifically, color, form, and number. These categories are presumably learned through an explicit reasoning process. The WCST is essentially a hypotheses-testing task in which the person being examined is presented with stimuli and must learn which stimuli belong to which category, presumably initially through a trial-and-error process. The person taking the test makes a response about category membership and then receives positive or negative feedback from the examiner in order to learn the categorical dimensions. So in order to perform well, the subject is required to discover the stimulus-based characteristics of the test, as was thoroughly discussed in the problem-solving paradigm discussed in *The Myth of Executive Functioning* [20]. This type of task activates not only the prefrontal cortex, but also the head of the caudate nucleus and other regions of the basal ganglia [14, 15]. Different brain regions are recruited during different phases of task administration; however, it is primarily considered a "frontal lobe" subtest. Although the Tower of London test is also a problem-solving task, it is not dependent upon rule-based category learning. The only commonality between the WCST and the TOL is that successful performance on both tasks is a function of the subject's ability to determine the stimulus-based characteristics of these measures. Again, the very vast range of "problem-solving" was the theme of volume II.

There are key differences between the administration of the WCST and the TOL. The examiner informs the examinee on correct and incorrect responses on the WCST, but offers no such input on the TOL. The examinee must determine when to adapt and adjust their problem solving strategy in regard to the changing demands of the task. While the examiner cannot prevent the subject from impulsive responding, this variable is not formally measured and can only be inferred from observation. On the TOL, the "planning time" variable is measured. Again, the TOL offers no examiner 'environmentally imposed structure' to the examinee. In this sense, the

WCST is a more structured task, while the TOL requires complete examinee self-direction and adjustment.

On the Tower of London test, the examinee is required to plan ahead and to organize thinking in order to determine the order of moves which are necessary to rearrange three colored beads which sit on pegs of descending length. The patient is required to work from an initial starting position which is always the same, in which the beads are placed on two of the three pegs, to move the beads to a new predetermined position with the beads on one or more of the pegs. The examinee is required to follow certain rules: only one bead may be moved at a time; all of the beads must be placed on a peg when they are not being moved; the number of beads that can be placed on any peg is specified by the length of the particular peg. This is technically a procedural rule-learning task, because the principle that underlies every item is exactly the same; however, the task is primarily used as a problem-solving measure, and not as a procedural-learning subtest as it is in much of the literature. Most of the literature applies different task variables, so it cannot be interpreted as a procedural learning task in its current format [16].

During completion of this task, the subject does not receive feedback from the examiner about his or her performance. The task presumably places heavy demands upon working memory functions, organizational and planning skills, and appropriate imagination for the purpose of the problem-solving. This task activates the dorsolateral prefrontal cortex, the anterior cingulate, the cuneus and the precuneus, and the cerebellum. Parietal lobe activation is observed in the supramarginal gyrus and angular gyrus. Activity has also been demonstrated within the basal ganglia, dependent upon the phase of the task. Therefore, this task activates a very complicated problem-solving network, although it does not activate the same types of networks that are activated by the WCST [17]. Based upon neuroanatomical concepts, one would not expect that these two tests would strongly correlate with each other; however, understanding the different dimensions of these tasks, along with their different neuroanatomical substrates, provides the examiner with considerable information that becomes synergistic when comparing performances of the two tasks together, in aggregate. Consider the following sets of scores which compare one 16 year old male patient's performance on the Wisconsin Card Sorting Test and the Tower of London test:

Test results

WCST	Raw scores	Age-corrected Standard scores	T-scores	%iles
Trials administered	74			
Total correct	66			
Total errors	8	124		95th
% Errors				
Perseverative responses	5	127		96th
% Perseverative responses				
Perseverative errors	5	126		96th

Test results

WCST	Raw scores	Age-corrected Standard scores	T-scores	%iles
% Perseverative errors				
Nonperseverative errors	3	121		92nd
% Nonperseverative errors				
Conceptual level responses				
% Conceptual level responses	89 %	126		96th
Categories completed	6			>16th
Trials to complete 1st category	11			>16th
Failure to maintain set	1			>16th
Learning to learn				

Test results

TOL	Raw	Age-corrected Standard scores	%iles
Initial move time	58″	106	66th
Problems correct	2	86	18th
Total moves	54	72	3rd
Execution time	356″	68	2nd
Total time	414″	70	2nd
Time violations	2	68	2nd
Errors	0	104	61st

After being administered two different problem-solving tasks, which are presumably dependent upon "frontal lobe" functions, the data appear contradictory. The patient's performance on the WCST is not only well within normal limits, but is within the "very-to-extremely high range" in comparison with same-age peers. On the other hand, the results of the TOL test may be best described as considerably poorer than expected. This patient was a "good" problem-solver on the WCST, but proved to be extremely poor at problem-solving on the TOL test. Why did this occur, and what can be learned from this example? Sufficient information has been provided in the introduction of both of these tasks; however, the overall conclusion can be greatly simplified and made extremely practical for interpretive purposes once the examiner is aware of the substrates of these tests.

On the Tower of London test, this individual used just about as much "planning time" as anyone else in attempting to think through solutions to problems before initiating a behavioral response. Therefore, an impulsive problem-solving approach was not identified, but the reader is cautioned: always review the initial item response times. We often observe patients that spend much time before responding to just one TOL item, which inflates the First Move score, while perhaps the cumulative First Move Time was very low across the other nine problems.

Poor problem-solving ability was noted (above) in the number of total moves this individual required to solve the problems, and in the number of items the individual solved in the minimum number of moves. First, the Total Move score at the third percentile ranking should be used as a statistical "marker." Once again, this test does not follow the normal distribution of a bell-shaped curve; therefore, there is nothing "very low" or "borderline" about this individual's performance. In other words, the individual's Total Move score at the third percentile says that this individual's problem-solving capability is poor. Nevertheless, the results of these two tests should be compared in aggregate so that a synergistic interpretation emerges.

On the WCST, the patient is given feedback about the accuracy of his or her performance on a trial-by-trial basis. Category membership is determined through the provision of constant and explicit feedback regarding the individual's responding, telling the individual whether each response was right or wrong immediately after each response. Therefore, results of the WCST indicate this particular patient was attentive to and responsive to informational feedback, and that with sufficient structure (i.e., being informed of the accuracy of each response as he made each response) he was able to perform quite well. Conversely, when that structure was removed during the TOL and the patient was required to maintain several rules in mind while developing a solution or procedure for solving the problem, the patient proved to have significant difficulty managing this type of ambiguity. Therefore, the conclusion is offered that this individual functions well in structured, routine, predictable situations; however, when confronted with novel circumstances that do not provide clues about successful performance, this individual, even though he took time to engage in planning and organization, was unable to effectively apply information to successfully solve the TOL problems on his own (i.e., without feedback from the examiner). This type of disparity has also been reported by Podell and colleagues [18].

One might predict that in structured and predictable circumstances, the types of situations that are inherent within a daily routine, this individual would not demonstrate any obvious deficiencies in functioning; however, when required to use independent judgment in decision-making, he would have notable difficulty in arriving at appropriate adaptive decisions. This patient's case demonstrates that data from the WCST and TOL proved to be diagnostically and practically synergistic. Had the results of the WCST been used in isolation, it would be difficult to ascertain much about this individual. Similarly, using the results of the TOL test in isolation would indicate this individual has difficulty with problem solving, but again would not provide as much clinically and diagnostically relevant information as synergistic pattern analysis of both tests. By understanding the underpinnings of both of these tasks, and by then comparing one performance to another, we learned much more about this patient than we would have learned had we examined each test result in isolation.

Theoretically, this type of synergistic information is useful for treatment planning. For example, the data imply that this individual would function at his very best in structured circumstances. Therefore, any treatment strategies that are devised to help this person, even without knowing the specific referral question, probably include a high degree of environmentally imposed structure as this individual is structure-dependent. When this individual is on his own, with little organization being imposed upon his life, he likely experiences difficulties in making adaptive decisions. Simply put, it is likely that his judgment cannot be trusted when functioning on an independent, autonomous basis in novel situations that in a sense "do not tell him what to do". Of course, this conclusion might seem over-arching because we presented so little information about this person; however, this inference is derived in order to assist the reader in understanding how relevant test scores can be used in a synergistic manner. The underlying and most critical points are the comparison of one relevant measure to another relevant measure within the same general dimension of functioning.

Summary

This chapter reviewed the interpretation of learning and memory tests and certain tests of "problem-solving." We hope we fulfilled several purposes. One purpose was to introduce the closely related individual comparison standard and the pattern analysis approaches of test interpretation. In the process of our interpretations, we demonstrated how certain statistically derived scores and comparisons within a simple "level of performance" group norm are inappropriate. We have demonstrated how certain categorizations of scores into statistically derived terminology can be contradictory and misleading. We have similarly illustrated the power of these methods of interpreting test data by referring to the synergistic conclusions that can emerge from the data. We have also revealed how in many instances, knowing about a person's "raw scores" are very powerful indicators of functioning and how statistical transformations are unnecessary in certain circumstances. Finally, we stressed the importance of knowing about how tests are constructed and standardized, as well as knowing about the neuro-biologic substrates of tests are always critical to test interpretation because this informs us diagnostically and leads to treatment planning.

References

1. Squire, L. R., & Shimamura, A. P. (1996). The neuropsychology of memory dysfunction and its assessment. In I. Grant & K. Adams (Eds.), *Neuropsychological assessment of neuropsychiatric disorders* (pp. 232–262). New York, NY: Oxford University Press.
2. Eichenbaum, H. (2010). Memory systems. *WIREs Cognitive Science, 1*, 478–490. doi:10.1002/wcs.49.
3. Squire, L. R., & Shimamura, A. P. (1996). The neuropsychology of memory dysfunction and its assessment. In I. Grant & K. Adams (Eds.), *Neuropsychological assessment of neuropsychiatric disorders* (pp. 232–262). New York, NY: Oxford University Press.
4. Lichter, D. G., & Cummings, J. L. (2001). *Frontal-subcortical circuits in psychiatric and neurological disorders*. New York, NY: The Guilford Press.
5. Delis, D. C., Kramer, J. H., Kaplan, E., & Ober, B. A. (2000). *California verbal learning test* (2nd ed.). San Antonio, TX: Psychological Corporation.

6. Simons, J. S., & Spiers, H. J. (2003). Prefrontal and medial temporal lobe interactions in long-term memory. *Nature Neuroscience Review, 4*, 637–648.

7. Salmon, D. P., & Bondi, M. W. (2009). Neuropsychological assessment of dementia. *Annual Review of Psychology, 60*, 257–282.

8. Wechsler, D. (2009). *Wechsler memory scale* (4th ed.). San Antonio, TX: Pearson.

9. Fuster, J. M. (2008). *The prefrontal cortex* (4th ed.). London, England: Academic Press.

10. Stuss, D. T. (2007). New approaches to prefrontal lobe testing. In B. L. Miller & J. L. Cummings (Eds.), *The human, frontal lobes: Functions and disorders* (2nd ed., pp. 292–305). New York, NY: Guilford Press.

11. Osterrieth, P. (1944). Le test de copie d'une figure complexe. *Archieves de Psychologie, 30*, 206–356.

12. Hoffmann, M. (2013). The human frontal lobes and frontal network systems: An evolutionary, clinical, and treatment perspective. *ISRN Neurology, 2013*, 892459.

13. Kent, J. (2013). The evolution of the Wechsler Memory Scale: A selective review. *Applied Neuropsychology Adult, 20*(4), 277–291.

14. Koziol, L. F., & Budding, D. E. (2009). *Subcortical structures and cognition: Implications for neuropsychological assessment*. New York, NY: Springer.

15. Mirsky, A. F. (1996). Disorders of attention: A neuropsychological perspective. In G. R. Lyon & N. A. Krasnegor (Eds.), *Attention, memory, and executive function* (pp. 71–95). Baltimore, MD: Paul H. Brookes.

16. Beauchamp, M. H., Dagher, A., Aston, J. A., & Doyon, J. (2003). Dynamic functional changes associated with cognitive skill learning of an adapted version of the Tower of London task. *NeuroImage, 20*, 1649–1660.

17. Best, J. R., & Miller, P. H. (2010). A developmental perspective on executive function. *Child Development, 81*(6), 1641–1660. http://doi.org/10.1111/j.1467-8624.2010.01499.x.

18. Podell, K., Lovell, M., & Goldberg, E. (2001). Lateralization of frontal lobe functions. In S. Salloway, P. Malloy, & J. Duffy (Eds.), *The frontal lopes and neuropsychiatric illness* (pp. 83–100). Washington, DC: American Psychiatric.

19. Koziol, L. F., Budding, D. E., & Chidekel, D. (2013). *ADHD as a model of brain-behavior relationships*. New York, NY: Springer.

20. Koziol, L. F. (2014). *The myth of executive functioning: Missing elements in conceptualization, evaluation, and assessment*. New York, NY: Springer.

Chapter 5
The Interpretive Significance of Pathognomonic Signs

"Any fact facing us is not as important as our attitude toward it, for that determines our success or failure."

Norman Vincent Peale

"I don't believe in psychology. I believe in good moves."

Robert James Fischer

There are a number of behaviors that are almost always clinically relevant and diag-nostically significant. These behaviors are usually observed infrequently, depending upon the age of the person being evaluated and the pathology in question. Reitan, when initially examining adult populations, originally referred to these behaviors as "pathognomonic" signs of impairment [1]. None of these pathognomonic behaviors follow the standardized normal distribution of a bell-shaped curve or any of the assumptions which support statistical quantification. Pathognomonic signs follow a *dichotomous distribution* and are often more within the realm of "have-have not" observations. The *INS DICTIONARY OF NEUROPSYCHOLOGY* defines pathog-nomonic signs as "findings that are specific for a given disease and that are not associated with other conditions" [2]. The term originally referred to characteristic behaviors observed in specific disease processes, and, outside the context of specific diseases, pathognomonic signs have *not* been well studied in pediatric populations with neuro-developmental disorders.

Clinical neuropsychology would be a perfect, exact science if there were norma-tive data for both clinical and normal control group populations. And it would be ideal if these data extended throughout the age range for which any given test would apply [3]. Furthermore, almost absolute perfection would be achieved in the field if every test was specifically linked to practical behaviors that could be observed out-side of the practitioner's office, in "real world" settings. However, in reality, nothing could be further from the truth, and the ecological validity of neuropsychological testing has been questioned [4]. In clinical neuropsychology, there is a relative

© Springer International Publishing Switzerland 2016

L.F. Koziol et al., *Large-Scale Brain Systems and Neuropsychological Testing* , DOI 10.1007/978-3-319-28222-0_5 absence of these ecologically valid test data; a practitioner's clinical judgment is necessary. Test results simply must be examined from a qualitative point of view, and this includes considering specific behavioral observations of abnormality; when such behaviors are identified, in and of themselves, they are major indicators of dysfunction, or "pathognomonic signs" of impairment. In pediatric populations with developmental disorders the children likely to arrive in the out-patient practitioner's office frequently require the generation of inferential conclusions that are not described in any diagnostic "cook book." Clinical judgment is definitely required for neuropsychological interpretations that are ecologically valid. These interpretations often seem dependent upon intuition that develops slowly from the accumulation of the clinician's experience. But this "intuitive judgment," known as information integration category learning, has been formally investigated. A neuro-biologic substrate supports this type of clinical intuition [5–7]. In our opinion, perhaps as a general rule of thumb, test interpretations that do not predict, or are not consistent with "out-of-office" behaviors are useless! Yet there must be some systematic way to think about these observations to make neuropsychological, diagnostic, "common sense" inferences that are not haphazard guess work from one case presentation to another.

Just like any other methodology for making clinical inferences from diagnostic test data, the pathognomonic sign approach features its own set of pluses and minuses, or positive and negative characteristics. The observance of a pathognomonic behavior nearly always implies the same interpretation; it carries the same meaning in each and every instance. This reduces the likelihood of false positive and false negative error. The identification and interpretation of these "signs" actually supersedes test data interpretations based upon statistical transformations of scores on tests; it by-passes categorical terminologies such as "borderline, low average, or average, etc." which are "umbrella-like" categories that contribute little to our understanding of people. However, identifying pathognomonic data is dependent upon the knowledge base and experience of the examiner, especially in pediatric symptom identification and diagnosis. Because the experience levels of pediatric neuropsychologists differ widely, these signs might not be identified and/or interpreted in the same way by different clinicians [8]. Pathognomonic signs might not be present consistently, and they might not be demonstrated by every individual with any given disorder. Finally, in many instances, test publishers might "force" a pathognomonic sign from a highly skewed, dichotomous distribution into a percentile ranking band, which then might mask the appropriate significance of the behavior. This has been done with certain memory tests, go-no go tasks, and with some tasks of phonological processing, to name just a few simple examples. The application of any single method of clinical inference can lead to misinterpretation; it has always been proposed that using multiple levels of inferential analysis simultaneously, systematically, and interactively, as initially introduced by Reitan [9], generates the most meaningful, ecologically valid interpretations. Within that context, the identification of pathognomonic signs of impairment is a diagnostically powerful methodology.

The finger-to-nose test often administered during the course of a neurological examination provides a direct example of the identification and interpretation of a pathognomonic sign. This procedure only has four possible outcomes; a completely "normal" performance, which does not necessarily rule-out pathology; tremor; an "over-shooting" of the finger when attempting to point to the nose; or an "under-shooting" of the nose. Whenever error occurs, it implicates involvement of the cerebellum. Hence, this represents a specific, or pathognomonic, sign of dysfunction within the cerebellum. The neuro-biologic substrate of this test was explained in Ito's description of a cerebellar control model [10, 11]; also, see Koziol & Lutz [12] for review. In this particular case, the specific "sign" has both diagnostic and localization significance. Diagnostically, the inability to effectively execute the behavior indicates the patient is unable to adapt to the changing requirements of the movement, as they unfold in an ongoing way, which is necessary to touch the nose. The localization significance concerns the activation of a cerebellar control model during the execution of the movement. In this way, the neuro-biologic substrate of the behavior is at least putatively known and generally accepted. This test is not ordinarily used during the course of neuropsychological evaluation; however, there is absolutely no reason why it cannot be used when an examiner might suspect involvement of medial/intermediate regions of the cerebellum. The question then becomes, at what age should we expect a child to "pass" the finger-to-nose screening "test?" The adult neurological examination includes a variety of other behaviors, including certain abnormal reflexes that in each and every instance point toward a specific symptomatic identification and possibly specific neurologic disease process. Again, the underpinnings of the task are clinically understood; the finger-to-nose test has never been "normed" and has never been "revised" because those statistical concepts are irrelevant to the task. We propose there are certain neuropsychological tasks of pathognomonic significance in pediatric populations with neuro-developmental disorders that similarly do not require "norming" or "revision." Application of statistical procedures to tasks such as these "misses" the point of symptom identification and interpretation. Furthermore, the neuro-biologic substrates of these tasks are known. Most practitioners are not taught the pediatric neurological examination, so our discussion is limited to commonly used neuropsychological tests.

In adult clinical neuropsychology, there are a number of specific signs of pathognomonic significance. Perhaps the easiest sign to describe that is known to every clinician is disorientation. For example, as indicated previously, when an individual is disoriented to time, it means that the brain is no longer capable of keeping track of experience in a continuous manner. Therefore, disorientation implies brain-related pathology. It must be noted that disorientation itself may occur for a variety of reasons, and it can be observed in a variety of unrelated pathologies; therefore, a pathognomonic or specific sign of impairment does not necessarily always have localizing significance and it might not always point to a specific disease process. A similar statement may be made concerning disorientation to place; however, disorientation to time is considered the most sensitive index of pathology, followed by disorientation to place, which is then followed by the pathognomonic sign of disorientation to person [13]. These signs occur infrequently within the pediatric population, there is no universal agreement as to what age we should expect a child to be fully oriented, but disorientation is frequently seen in certain adult pathologies such as concussion, delirium and/or dementia [14]. It is generally accepted that the observance of these signs usually involves a diffuse type of neuro-anatomical substrate, although the specific pathology might be acute or chronic.

Aphasic symptoms and all of the agnosias are considered signs of pathognomonic significance in adult populations [15, 16]. These signs seldom occur in psychiatric populations, but they are observed with considerable frequency in patient populations with documented brain impairment that is usually severe. There are varieties of disease processes, most of them observed within young adults and/or adult and geriatric populations, which generate aphasia and agnosia which are of considerable pathognomonic diagnostic significance, but the authors we have cited present the most useful information, because those chapters focus upon symptom identification and neuro-anatomic substrates. These signs can be interpreted in a very literal fashion. The sign might not always have localizing significance, although these pathognomonic indicators always imply a brain-related pathology and/or some sort of neurologic disease process. Therefore, knowledge of pathognomonic signs represents a powerful diagnostic index for neuropsychologists.

False Positive and False Negative Errors

When certain cases lack clarity, over-use or misinterpretation of "pathognomonic signs" may lead to a greater likelihood of a false positive error. Some case presentations are inherently ambiguous. No diagnostic test or behavioral observation is perfect in any field. Any test can run the risk of "false positive" or "false negative" error. As a good rule of thumb to follow, an examiner should ask himself/herself the question of the risk factors associated with making a false positive versus making a false negative error because these possibilities always exist when there is interpretive uncertainty. For instance, in a possible dementia patient, calling a behavior pathognomonic of Alzheimer's disease has extremely negative implications for the patient, family, and for treatment, even if the level of impairment is relatively mild. In that case, the nomenclature of "mild cognitive impairment" (MCI) seems in order; qualifying statements should include the fact that a baseline of the person's cognitive functioning has been established for the purpose of future comparisons, and that approximately 5 % of MCI presentations convert to demonstrating more obvious signs of dementia after about a year [17]. However, in a child, the implications are considerably different. An examiner might feel much more comfortable when the likelihood of false positive error exists if the outcome can only lead to an early intervention that increases the likelihood of a good developmental outcome. Early interventions avoid wasting precious "intervention time," and no "harm" will be associated with the outcome. Therefore, the term "pathognomonic sign" should be used cautiously if there is any lack of clarity when evaluating a behavior or cognitive skill set. The examiner should be aware of the risks involved. When ambiguity exists, the astute practitioner is in a position of predicting possible risk outcomes, almost "picking" the type of error that might be made by associating this with likely future outcomes, while including the appropriate qualifying statements in the diagnostic report. In this way, the examiner is always acting in the best interest of the patient.

Pathognomonic Signs in Neuro-Developmental Disorders

Within the adult population, the identification of a pathognomonic sign is dependent upon an important assumption: the expectation is made that the specific or pathognomonic sign represents a loss of functioning from a level that was previously intact. Quite obviously, this assumption is problematic when attempting to identify pathognomonic signs within the developing pediatric population. A pediatric assessment is essentially evaluating a "moving target." For instance, at what age can we assume that any given facet of cognition or behavior has been acquired? Because of the developmental process, some clinicians argue that pathognomonic signs can only very rarely be identified within the pediatric population. Others may argue that a failure to acquire certain skills represents a pathognomonic or a specific sign of impairment. Within the population of young children, the term "developmental delay" is sometimes synonymous with "pathognomonic," with the former label being perhaps a bit more palatable to parents while respecting the dynamic nature of pediatric neurodevelopment. The specific age of acquisition of certain behaviors is not universally agreed upon, so the emergence of some behaviors is expected to occur within a certain "band" of age ranges. In many instances, the band of age ranges is extremely large, and this generates ambiguity and encourages a "wait and see" monitoring attitude. Therefore, during childhood, terming a behavior "pathognomonic" should be done with caution. To reiterate, pathognomonic implies brain-related impairment with certainty. The term "developmental delay" does not, and perhaps implies immature development. In our opinion, a behavior may be termed pathognomonic if it lies outside of the expectation of what is known about sensory, motor, and neurocognitive developmental milestones; however, there also are certain qualitative behaviors that can be interpreted with pathognomonic significance. For example, certain types of word mispronunciations, misarticulations, and grammatical errors are pathognomonic of language disorder.

On the other hand, if a patient's developmental history reveals behaviors that are highly predictive of pathological neuro-development, is it reasonable to term that very early occurring behavior pathognomonic? It certainly can be predictive of certain types of sensory, neurocognitive, or neurobehavioral impairment. For example, we have previously indicated that a neonate's failure to latch on and/or problems with sucking/swallowing cycles, are associated with an increased likelihood of developmental language disorders [18]. This is *predictive information; it tells us what is likely to occur down the developmental road. Technically, it is not a "pathognomonic sign" observed in a test protocol, either in terms of a test score or a qualitative observation.* Nevertheless, the fundamental fact of the matter is that specific pathognomonic signs that might emerge from test data have not been systematically studied within pediatric populations, so there are no universally agreed upon behaviors of specific significance for each and every practitioner. Therefore, two different practitioners might have two completely different diagnostic impressions about any given child.

Nevertheless, in our opinion, sufficient and well replicated test and behavioral data are now available to identify certain "signs" of pathognomonic significance that indicate specific symptoms in some neuro-developmental disorders. The neuro-anatomical underpinnings of these "signs" are known from systematic investigations. The sample of pathognomonic signs that are presented here carry minimal risk of "false positive" error. These specific signs follow a dichotomous distribution and they *should* always lead to an early intervention. This serves the purpose of providing a direct treatment that can never be harmful but instead, can only promote development. Finally, and perhaps most importantly, considering these observations as pathognomonic of deficit is very badly needed within the field because, in each and every instance, identification of these signs in neuro-developmental disorders avoids a "wait and see" approach, which we prefer to term a "wait and fail" policy, therefore avoiding a literal "waste of developmental time" in eventually providing intervention at a time that might already be too late, or at a period in development when only limited progress might be expected. Therefore, this position is completely defensible at a variety of levels. The first step in an achieving a general consensus or agreement can only serve to assist the field in moving forward.

Continuous Performance Tests, Stop Signal Tasks, and Go-No Go Paradigms: Unfortunate Misunderstandings and the Controversy

A discussion of the use of these tasks in diagnosing ADHD is bound to generate heated arguments in a room that contains only a handful of neuropsychologists! Every practitioner participating in the discussion might have a completely different opinion; however, at the risk of being considered "rogue" and/or at least stubborn and misleading, we have decided to go against our "best judgment" in our concerted effort to "set the matter straight," and our "opinionated arrogance" does not stop there! The goal is to achieve universal agreement on, perhaps, the most difficult issue we will be addressing. Obviously, none of us are immune to criticism, but in this case, a close examination of the controversy is welcomed. Whenever such ambiguity and lack of agreement exists, this must mean that the stimulus based properties of the issue are incompletely understood, and that the field of neuropsychology might have been asking the wrong questions. As stated in *The Myth of Executive Functioning* [27] of this series, it is time to pause, use our imagination, think, and propose a new set of questions; if these questions are answered by meeting the stimulus based properties of the ambiguity, this just might eliminate the "problem." Then again, perhaps our anticipation of "controversy" is actually a distorted prediction to begin with, in which case a revisiting of these paradigms provides a refreshing review. Establishing an anchor point provides a strong base to which we can return just in case an idea or two leads us astray in our navigation through these "troubled waters." Therefore, we are using continuous performance tests (CPTs), stop signal tasks, and go-no go paradigms to provide the anchor point—stability in terms of knowing where we started from. If this presentation does not lead us to "pathognomonic signs," then we can summarily dismiss our argument. Nothing lost, nothing gained, except perhaps breaking-up an otherwise completely boring day. It is blatantly clear that our biggest risk with respect to this section is an attempt at humor without knowing about the stimulus based character- istics of the reader our audience, who might not find our facetiousness appropriate for a clinical treatise!

There is no single neuropsychological "litmus test" for diagnosing ADHD [19, 20]. In fact, the Test of Variables of Attention (TOVA), arguably the first commer- cially available CPT, was never intended to serve as a "test" to diagnose ADHD [21]. Instead, the TOVA was designed to assist physicians in titrating psychostimu- lant medication dosage in individuals who were already diagnosed with ADHD according to the DSM behaviorally defined criteria. In fact, using the TOVA to make a diagnosis of ADHD in any given person is a misapplication of the test to begin with (see *ADHD as a Model of Brain-Behavior Relationships* [26]. for detailed review). This is not a subtle point; it is a major diagnostic issue that should be of concern to every practitioner. Furthermore, there are well over 200 CPTs described in the experimental and zclinical literature, while a "handful" of these different CPTs are available for commercial application [22]. None of these differ- ent CPT methodologies were developed for the purpose of diagnosing ADHD, nor do these paradigms measure the same clinical variables. No CPT should ever be used to diagnose ADHD; instead, to make that diagnosis, the behavioral observa- tions listed within the DSM are the critical variables of interest (Barkley, latest book addition, or previous book). Finally, broad-based neuropsychological test batteries have never reliably differentiated anyone with ADHD from those indi- viduals without the disorder, or any of the DSM subtypes of the disorder ([23, 24]; see Koziol & Stevens, [25], for additional review). The absolute best that can be hoped for is establishing a *correlation* between a test, or battery of tests, and a behaviorally defined diagnosis of ADHD. But this only tells us the frequency, or percentage of time that a diagnosis of ADHD co-occurs with a test/battery of tests.

The pediatric practitioner should not be interested in the percentage of time a test score, or a pattern of test scores, correlates with any given diagnosis. The clinical neuropsychologist, by definition, should be concerned with knowing about and iden- tifying brain-behavior relationships. In a comprehensive and detailed argument, Koziol, Budding, and Chidekel [26] described the differences between a DSM behav- iorally defined diagnosis and descriptive neuropsychological nomenclature. The DSM was not intended to meet the descriptive needs of neuropsychology; neuropsychology never intended to meet the diagnostic needs of the DSM. These are two completely different systems, but using these systems in combination provides synergistic infor- mation—the DSM generates a categorical diagnosis; neuropsychological assessment informs the clinician about the relevant brain-behavior relationships that are affected, and identifies the symptoms to be treated or managed (see *ADHD as a Model of Brain-Behavior Relationships* [26] for review). In the end, DSM disorders are treated symptomatically, and a comprehensive neuropsychological evaluation compliments the DSM by identifying the brain systems involved for any given patient. The DSM provides an over-arching diagnostic label, but all patients with the same diagnosis do not share the same symptom picture; neuropsychological evaluation differentiates the "drivers" of various symptoms and therefore "bridges the gap" between these two systematic approaches. The result is synergistic because the "product" provides information that would not be known by using either system in isolation. This is not at all the same as using tests to identify any specific disorder. Furthermore, there is no use for computer print-outs and/or neuropsychological reports that describe presumed *aspects of attention* as "mildly atypical" and/or resembling a clinical population with an attention problem to any stated statistically derived degree. Believe it or not, knowing about these differences is critical to deriving pathognomonic signs from CPTs, stop signal tasks, and go-no go paradigms. This augmentation of our anchor point should be understood so well by the practitioner that these issues become comfortable conversational dialogue or discourse before moving on to investigating the purposes of these test paradigms and their application in neuropsychological evaluation. This level of comprehension is absolutely necessary for applying these methodologies and interpreting the results they generate as "pathognomonic signs." If this deeper level of understanding has not yet been achieved, the reader is compelled to return to the anchor point for additional review.

It is incumbent upon the reader to concede that the topic of "attention" is an extremely vast area and to acknowledge that the fields of cognitive, academic-experimental, and neuropsychology all have very different considerations in mind when studying and understanding attention. These fields do not communicate well with each other. This is not to say that the fields of cognitive and academic psychology are irrelevant to the neuropsychology of attention [28, 29]. It does mean that in neuropsychological evaluation, elements of attention are examined selectively; however, a comprehensive presentation of the variables of attention relevant to all these fields is well beyond the scope of this volume series. We are primarily interested in presenting information of clinical application. In this regard, the first CPT was developed to measure sustained attention and vigilance [30]. This task was not dependent upon the span of attention within a mnemonic dimension as might be inferred from a Digit Span subtest, nor was it dependent upon the internally driven speed and visual search of cancellation-type tasks, even though these tasks might require a type of "sustained performance." Instead, the original CPT placed a limited stimulus load on the subject, with minimal cognitive demand, but nevertheless making attention difficult to sustain because of its repetitive, lengthy nature. The task was simple and of little interest to the subject; a button was to be pressed when a certain target letter (such as an "A") was observed, but only when this target letter was presented after another anticipatory stimulus (the letter "A" after the letter "X"). In this way, the subject taking the test was responsible for correctly identifying correct stimulus presentations and to "not respond" or inhibit responses to other stimuli, such as the "alerting" or anticipatory stimuli. The number of total stimuli presented was controlled, the rate of stimulus presentations/interstimulus interval was held constant, and obviously the memory load of the task was minimal, *primarily because test performance is sensitive to these variables*. This test was administered to a wide range of subjects from children (a preschool version of the task) through adulthood. *Under these circumstances, with all of the above described variables controlled, errors of omission (failing to identify a stimulus) and errors of commission (responding to an anticipatory stimulus or other stimuli that required inhibition) never, ever followed the normal distribution of a bell-shaped curve; errors were very minimal in children as young as 4 years of age and throughout adulthood, following a highly skewed distribution at all ages* (although errors followed a developmental trajectory, the discussion of which goes well beyond the scope of this chapter (the interested reader is referred to Stevens, et al., [31])). This means that subjects who made more numerous errors exhibited disturbed attentional functions. In other words, errors were **pathognomonic of deficit** (Mirsky, personal communication, 2008; [30]).

As neuro-diagnostic methodologies became more advanced, our knowledge of the various elements of attention slowly developed. The brain structures and neural networks that constitute the neuro-anatomic substrates of attentional systems became increasingly clear [32, 33]. The composition of the tasks applied to evaluate attention became better understood. Some of these "data" are both revealing and surprising. Although it is very tempting to review all of these variables, this manuscript is restricted to a discussion of only those factors relevant to CPT and inhibition paradigms; other variables were reviewed in Volume I of this series [26]. Similarly, Koziol, Joyce, and Wurglitz [34] revisited and updated what has been referred to as the "Mirsky model of attention," a systematic, practical approach to the neuropsychological assessment of attention, which included a current review of the neuro-anatomic substrates of the various dissociable component processes of attention.

In any event, the fact that all commercially available CPTs are not alike and do not allow for "pathognomonic sign" inferences is critical to our current discussion. The CPT is clinically relevant only if it is constructed according to the methodology originally proposed by Rosvold and colleagues [30, 35–39]. To our knowledge, the Gordon Diagnostic System is the only available CPT that mimics this methodology [40]. The CPT developed by Rosvold and colleagues, and which was subsequently computerized by Mirsky, was never made available through the commercial market. This methodology is vital because, as it turns out, the right hemisphere frontal-parietal network (FPN) supports this type of CPT performance. When "targets" immediately following an anticipatory, alerting stimulus are presented relatively rarely, in the neighborhood of only 11 % of the time [41], the burden of withholding responses, or response inhibition as assessed by commission errors, is under the control of the right hemisphere, ventral, frontal-striatal-pallidal-thalamo-cortical modulatory "loop" [42–44]. Neuro-imaging data also implicate the *indirect pathway* in a perhaps more specific brain-behavior relationship [31].

When target rate presentations increase to 25 % of the time, errors of commission substantially decline, and when target frequency is set at 50 %, there is a virtual absence of these errors. This occurs because targets are presented so frequently that the subject is responding too often—almost always, so that "frontal inhibition" is literally not required [41]. The right hemisphere ventral frontal network is not recruited, and presumably, this would specifically impact upon the "no-go" function of the indirect pathway. Many commercially available CPTs significantly increase and decrease the rate and number of target presentations, and in this way, it is virtually impossible to determine what is being evaluated; as a result, errors, or even their absence, can no longer be considered "pathognomonic signs" of anything! Changing target "numbers" of presentation and rate of presentation alters the interplay or interaction within the right hemisphere frontal-parietal system, or FPN. This system is preferentially connected to function as a "novelty detector" [45]. Its functional specialization profile is the substrate for "behavioral selections" driven by the external environment which is necessary for identifying and orienting to task *novelty* [46]. By definition, infrequently occurring stimuli or events are "novel." Without controlling for stimulus frequency and rate, the purpose of the CPT is defeated because the right hemisphere FPN is no longer predictably taxed or stressed; however, with rarely occurring presentations, the task remains novel, the cognitive demand for alertness and "control"(inhibition) are constant throughout the task, and because an efficient, intact FPN should not fail to detect novelty or respond to context prematurely, errors of omission and commission become "pathognomonic" of deficit. Furthermore, stop signal and go-no go tasks both require rarely occurring stimulus detection and inhibition, and therefore recruit the right hemisphere FPN as well. As conceptualized by Denckla and Reiss [47], dysfunction within the right hemisphere frontal-striatal system is evident when external sensory inputs that should trigger an action fail to do so (errors of omission), and inputs that should not be acted upon do trigger action (errors of commission/defective response inhibition). The more specific characteristics of stop signal and go-no go tasks are different from each other and from CPTs, but space requirements disallow this review; however, we fall back on Denckla and Reiss [47], who describe these tasks as requiring alertness and inhibition as critical factors for adjusting to the changing demands of these tasks as they develop or unfold.

So, what do CPTs, stop signal tasks, and go-no go task performances have to do with diagnosing ADHD? Absolutely nothing! However, these tasks, when constructed in a useful way, and when applied for the appropriate purpose, identify deficits in alertness and/or deficits in response inhibition. Lapses in attention or alertness activate the Default Mode Network or DMN, and this presumably means that attention is wandering and the individual is thinking about something other than the task at hand [33, 48]. Disinhibition, or errors of commission, reveal that the individual responded to a distracting stimulus and therefore might be termed "distractible" [31]. Identification of these symptoms, and in particular the "disinhibition" that generates distractibility, often predicts a positive response to treatment with psychostimulant medication [49–54] Similarly, errors made on a CPT when targets occur infrequently often correspond with complaints of forgetfulness [41]. Therefore, these "pathognomonic signs" *identify symptoms and behaviors that can be both predicted and treated, providing information that should be the ultimate goal of neuropsychological evaluation.* But without knowing about how a test was constructed, and without knowing the neuroanatomic substrates that support test performances and that can generate symptoms, neuropsychological evaluation is in a weak position, simply reduced to using tests that can only tell us how frequently a certain test performance co-occurs with any given DSM diagnosis. Unfortunately, the "tests" are no longer powerful tools, and with this relatively lengthy discussion, we are comfortable in believing that we have identified the "stimulus-based" properties of the controversy over misapplying these paradigms for "diagnosing" ADHD, while demonstrating the constructive application of these paradigms by identifying pathognomonic signs and their relationship to ecological validity. Hopefully, we have put the "neuro" back into the field of "neuropsychology." And this is perhaps best demonstrated by two, brief case examples.

Case 5

This is a case of a 12 year old boy who obtained the following scores on the Vigilance Task of the GDS:

	Raw	Percentile
GDS vigilance correct responses	41	20
GDS vigilance commission errors[a]	9	6
NEPSY knock and tap	–	11–25

All errors were to alerting stimuli.

Our interpretation here is obvious. According to the skewed performance profile of the norms for the GDS system, this seventh grader is both inattentive and distractible. And it is also notable that on "Knock and Tap," a type of go-no go paradigm, some readers might interpret that this performance falls within either the broad limits of average, or at best, within the "borderline" statistical category. However, we introduced this case fragment to illustrate a point. *Errors on go-no go paradigms do not follow a standardized normal distribution. The distribution is highly skewed, and a statistical transformation to a standard score of 90, equivalent to the 25th %ile, does not make the score "average." Broadening the band to encompass the 11th %ile similarly does not do justice to the data, perhaps referring to a "borderline" range. Not only are these over-arching categorical terms confusing, but they lack meaning. In a statistical transformation of a dichotomous distribution, when the most significant proportion of children are performing at the 50th %ile ranking or better, a score between the 11th and 25th %ile band is pathognomonic of deficit.* It is true that percentile rankings make huge differentiations based upon small normally distributed differences, but when tasks are "pathognomonic," characterized by errors that occur very rarely, that is exactly the point to be made. These tests of pathognomonic significance are simple, and they are constructed so that they do not tolerate very much error! As previously stated, the right hemisphere, ventral, frontal-striatal-pallidal-thalamo-cortical modulatory "loop" is implicated.

Case 6

This vignette concerns a Caucasian 7 year old female who was seen on multiple occasions for follow-up and to assist in updating her treatment plan. She presents with rather unique neurologic pathology. For example, her MRI findings include an absence of the cerebellar vermis, a fusion of the cerebellar hemispheres, and an absence of the primary fissure of the cerebellum. She was eventually diagnosed with the very rare disorder termed Gomez-Lopez-Hernandez Syndrome. We will return to this case in the next chapter, both for reviewing case history and to illustrate how test procedures can be modified to obtain additional "results" in order to demonstrate some of the functions of the cerebellum. However, for now, reviewing only her GDS Vigilance findings will suffice to uncover another important point.

	Raw	Percentile
GDS vigilance correct responses	39	65
GDS vigilance commission errors[a]	9	26

aAll errors, except one, were responses to alerting stimuli.

Several important issues emerge from reviewing even these limited data. First, it is definitely possible to separate errors of omission from errors of commission. These two error types have completely different meanings. This is because alertness and disinhibition are entirely different processes. This young girl was obviously alert. She was at least just as aware of the stimulus presentations on this task as anyone else within her peer group, so "paying attention" was not an issue. Nobody can argue about the reasonability of a score at the 65th percentile ranking, especially on a test of pathognomonic interpretative significance. She made *fewer* errors of omission than her peers! We previously indicated that the right hemisphere FPN is particularly involved in supporting performance on this task, and this level of alertness is likely a manifestation of an intact, functional right hemisphere parietal lobe. Second, because errors of commission never follow a normal distribution at any age, these data can be interpreted as demonstrating the dissociation of function between "posterior" and "anterior" frontal system regions, and with these errors at the 26th percentile, who is willing to quibble about using this "artificial, arbitrary score" as a pathognomonic sign? Third, once again, because commission errors always implicate involvement of the right hemisphere, ventral, frontal-striatal system, the data implicate that this system is involved in this case as well; however, this case fragment was presented specifically because of the objective, well documented pathology of the cerebellum. It is almost universally accepted that the cerebellum is an anticipatory control functional mechanism (please refer to *ADHD as a Model of Brain-Behavior Relationships* [26] and *The Myth of Executive Functioning* [27]. of this series for comprehensive reviews). For this case, as well as the previous case, both raise questions as to whether or not there is a cerebellar contribution to CPT performance, with perhaps a specific role in anticipatory control (The functional neuro-anatomical connectional profiles of both the frontal-striatal and the cerebro-cerebellar systems were also reviewed in the previously mentioned volumes *ADHD as a Model of Brain-Behavior Relationships* [26], which presented the symptoms of ADHD as a model of brain-behavior relationships, reviewed the role of the cerebellum in attention and in ADHD. *The Myth of Executive Functioning* [27] described how the entire vertebrate and human brain functions as a "prediction" mechanism in order to support Executive Functioning; however, to our knowledge, the cerebellum has only rarely been a region of interest in functional neuro-imaging investigations of patterns of brain area recruitment while performing a CPT [56, 57]. Therefore, the test data generated very useful information for identifying certain problematic symptoms such as distractibility. The results suggested at least one potentially viable treatment option, and the underlying neuro-anatomic underpinnings are presumably known; however, this does not at all mean that our knowledge of the symptoms of distractibility and all of its neuro-biologic substrates are completely identified and understood.

Reading and Spelling: Predictive Observations and Pathognomonic Signs of Disorder

Reading is, first and foremost, a language-based skill. It is an extension of the language system, and when things "go wrong" in the learning to read process, it is most often a manifestation of a deficit within the language system [58]. There are some exceptions, but overall, with respect to *dyslexia, which is defined as "a reading difficulty that is unexpected for a person's age, intelligence, level of education, or profession"* [59], reading disorder occurs because of systemic language based problems. Language supports reading ability, which is to say, reading is *parasitic* upon language [60]. When an English-speaking child is learning to read, the "message" given to the brain goes something like this: "Everything you heard, and everything you said in your previous years, can be transcribed into this system of symbols." So without the spoken word, or language, there would be absolutely nothing to transcribe!

Reading is not only of interest to us, but we are passionate about it. Reading underpins every academic subject any individual will ever pursue; it allows the individual to grow and develop within her/his profession. It helps us relax, perhaps as we read a fictitious novel. It allows us to understand the documentary books about the flight of APOLLO 13, which was an exceptional illustration of executive functioning in action. There is a very considerable literature about reading. We would love to write a book about the learning to read process, what can "go wrong," and how to remediate the problem. But once again, unfortunately, this is not our task in this volume; we are compelled to discuss pathognomonic signs. In today's neuropsychology, it is incumbent upon every practitioner to understand, identify, and interpret them.

Because reading is supported by language skills, knowing the developmental history about any given child's language functioning might provide valuable information about that particular child's reading development. Of course, this is unequivocally true; however, because there are such huge "windows" in developmental processes for such a wide range of reasons, developmental behavioral observations should absolutely never be used as a "cookbook" for predicting problems in the learning to read process. We have already stated that an infant's failure to "latch on" for breast feeding increases the likelihood for developmental language problems [18], and a delay in speaking can be the first clue that portends a later reading problem [59]. Similarly, speech is a "special instance" of a *motor skill*. In this regard, developmental motor anomalies can be a harbinger of learning to read problems when the child reaches school-age. Some of us might recall the "un-referenced" saying we might have been taught when we were in graduate-level training, specifically, "late to walk=late to talk=late to read."

ADHD as a Model of Brain-Behavior Relationships [26] and *The Myth of Executive Functioning* [28], and Koziol and Lutz [12] emphasized the necessity of understanding "bottom-up" development for truly appreciating the significant and ongoing contributions of subcortical structures and functions to "higher-level" cognitive processes. In this regard, if a child's behaviors are generated by maturational lags in cerebellar development during the course of early childhood, a characteristic pattern often unfolds [61–64]. This is manifest by relatively mild motor difficulty; the child is slower to sit-up independently and in walking without assistance. There can be an identification of the symptom of low muscle tone/hypotonia, which characteristically leads to problems with fine muscular and motor control. Because expressive language/speech production requires fine *oromotor control* over the speech musculature [65] for the purpose of proper articulation, as well as fine oromotor sequencing in the service of making speech sound-oromotor associations, developmental anomalies within these aspects of the language system can easily generate phonological processing deficits—which are a critical underpinning for reading. More conscious effort would then be necessary to accomplish "reading-related" tasks because of even subtle motor difficulties, reading-related tasks would be performed slowly, while in aggregate, the diminished allocation of cognitive resources/more effortful cognitive processing would take an additional toll on reading automaticity and comprehension. But all of these functions and processes are observations with a predictive character; these observations enable the clinician to understand language and reading development; they are not pathognomonic signs that indirectly identify reading disorder. Instead, these are risk factors that serve to predict an increased likelihood of a future diagnosis of dyslexia. This is a critical distinction.

Other similar risk factors include early color and/or letter identification problems that a parent might describe while reporting their child's history; in neuropsychological evaluation, numerous "tests" can be administered so that the practitioner can formally assess these behaviors, in which case they can be referred to as pathognomonic signs in school-aged children. Naming the letters of the alphabet, the names of colors, the names of numbers, or the names of common objects are all risk factors for reading difficulties in pre-school children [66]. At the time of school entry into the first grade, these behaviors should be thought about as pathognomonic signs of dyslexia, and they should be formally identified and quantified at least for the purpose of establishing a cognitive baseline. All of these observations are presumably dependent upon the same neuro-anatomic frontal-striatal retrieval mechanism and are really a manifestation of a language problem—another illustration of how the learning to read process is parasitic upon the language system. Other observations that are considered risk factors include letter-sound associations, such as asking the child to identify which word in a group has a different starting letter, for example, "boat-ball-and doll." Parents often "play" these types of word and/or rhyming "games" with their children, for example, "tell me a word that sounds the same as 'bat.'" These types of sound-word association "games" require speech-sound awareness, precursors of the phoneme and/or phonological processing that is more formally assessed during the course of neuropsychological evaluation. Just so long as hearing is intact, performance on these tasks is presumably dependent upon the integrity of Frontal-Parietal Networks; however, dependent upon the specific task, numerous other brain regions can be recruited, characterized by changing patterns of functional connectivity in both the left and right cerebral hemispheres [67, 68].

There are several language tasks that separate good readers from poor readers [69]. These tasks are speech perception, assessed by the ability to discriminate speech sounds from environmental sounds under less than optimal conditions; Productive vocabulary, essentially defined as object naming; Phonetic working memory problems; and deficits in syntax and/or semantics; however, the two most powerful predictors of Reading Disability are deficits in phoneme awareness and deficits in continuous rapid object naming. Phoneme awareness is characterized by a sensitivity to phonemes, which are the smallest sounds of speech, and deficiencies in this area are a major factor in reading disability. Phonological awareness includes sensitivity to rhyme, syllables, and morphemes, which are the smallest units of speech sounds that represent meaning, such as the "ea" in heal or health, or the "relat" in words of similar meaning such as relation, relationship, or relative. Most commercially available tasks combine phoneme with phonological awareness, but do not further complicate matters by including morphological awareness; however, it is important to be aware of these differences because isolated deficits in these areas might be observed in analyzing any given child's reading and/or spelling errors. The "double deficit" hypotheses of Reading Disorder is generally accepted according to Miller and colleagues [70]. This "double deficit" hypothesis is consistent with the two most common deficits in reading disorders, namely, deficits in both phonological processing and in continuous rapid object naming, which we consider pathognomonic signs of reading disorder. Children with reading disorder do not necessarily demonstrate deficits in both areas; however, those with only phonological processing deficits are remediated more easily than those with rapid object naming deficits. Those with only rapid naming deficits remediate more easily than those with deficits in both areas [71]. Therefore, assessing these functions independently is useful for both identifying reading disorder, for providing clues to understanding why a child cannot read, as well as for generating rough estimates about prognostic outcomes. (What we have summarized here are other summaries of a voluminous literature; the clinician attempting to diagnose reading disorders should be familiar with this vast literature.)

Because we acquire language using "whole words," it is understandable that subtle deficits in language processing might not be evident until a child is school-aged. So, what is it that makes phonemic and phonological awareness so important to learning how to read? Phonemic sensitivity is equivalent to saying the child is aware that "whole words" can be broken down to small speech sounds; phonological sensitivity corresponds to saying that whole words can be "broken down" into smaller "chunks," primarily referring to syllables. This knowledge, or "skill set," is never, ever required when children speak in whole words, phrases, and/or sentences. For a child to understand how the alphabet *really works,* letters, and certain groups of letters, must be associated or "matched" with the appropriate sounds. So, breaking whole words down into smaller sounds is absolutely necessary to link or "map" these sounds with the alphabet; unfortunately, the way we "sound out" letters of the alphabet is not the same as how these letters are used to associate sounds in words. Although there are 26 letters of the alphabet, the English language employs more than a thousand syllables! So learning these sound- symbol correspondences seems to pose a daunting task. To learn this "system," it is first necessary to be sensitive to the fact that words can be broken down into smaller units, and only then can any given child become aware of the relationship between printed and spoken words [69]. This explains a critical underpinning, and this type of knowledge is not something that we ever use in the usual, routine activities of listening and talking. Therefore, it has to be assessed formally, and, it is a pathognomonic sign because of the characteristics of its skewed distribution.

For example, 4, 5, and 6 year old children were required to indicate how many different sounds they could identify within a word by "tapping out" the number of sounds. None of the 4 year old children could tap the number of phonemes, although half of the group could tap the number of syllables. In the 5 year old group, 17 % of the children correctly tapped out the number of phonemes, and once again, about 50 % of the group correctly tapped the number of syllables within a word. However, in the 6 year old group, 70 % were able to tap the number of phonemes, and 90 % of that group correctly tapped syllables [72]. Therefore, syllabic identification develops before phoneme awareness, and between the ages of 4–6 years old, these underpinnings for reading develop very rapidly. Furthermore, the trajectory of the development of these abilities certainly does not follow the assumptions of a normal distribution, but instead, the distribution is highly skewed. This enables the practitioner to interpret phonological processing as a pathognomonic sign by the time a child reaches school-age and begins to learn to read within the classroom. Furthermore, as Mann and Liberman demonstrated, 85 % of children in kindergarten who went on to become good readers a year later in first grade correctly counted the numbers of syllables in spoken words [73] These data are persuasive, and following these basic guidelines, the chances of making a "false negative" error are minimal; any possible "false positive" error would be rare, and arguably can never lead to an intervention that would not be beneficial to any child.

Why should continuous rapid naming be associated with reading ability? In our opinion, the first reason is obvious! Reading is primarily "automatic." When two and three letter-words are learned, they become automatic as the typically developing child continuously reads them through no more than the ordinary repetition or "practice" inherent in the learning process. An additional reason is perhaps more subtle.

Reading requires associations between symbols and smaller speech sounds. Therefore, this might conceivably be understood as the "speed" with which a child acquires these associations, and this is related to reading fluency. When reading and words have been automated, the "brain" is literally engaged in a retrieval process, and in theory, this process is the same, if not highly similar, to general language word retrieval functions. In this way, the speed of "label" retrieval is the function identified. Wolf [74] and Mann [75] have both provided evidence that continuous naming tests of colors, objects, and letters are predictive of early problems in the learning to read process and that these are persistent problems observed in the test protocols of impaired readers [74, 75]. Although some might argue that slow naming speed is a special instance of generalized "slow processing speed," Bowers and Ishaik [71] concluded that slow naming speed is a factor that is independent or dissociated from other factors such as phonemic awareness and from the working memory "speed-accuracy trade-off"[76].

Reading disorder can also be identified by observing the child's reading and spelling errors. The characteristics of these errors imply a problem with integrating the phonological information that the sequences of letters convey. The child is very often able to pronounce the first letter in a word correctly, but they experience considerable difficulty with the subsequent letters in a word. Particular difficulties are noted with vowels as opposed to consonants [60]. In our opinion, these errors should be considered a pathognomonic sign of reading and or/spelling deficit, since practically every child with dyslexia also has a spelling problem. The following case vignette reveals "pathognomonic signs" in every area described above:

Case Sample: This patient is a 9 year old girl who was evaluated approximately 1 month before entering the fourth grade:

	Scaled/Standard score	Percentile rank
NEPSY phonological processing	8	25
NEPSY object naming	8	25
Accuracy	–	>75
Speed	–	11–25
WIAT II word reading	88	21
WIAT II pseudoword decoding	88	21
WIAT II spelling	73	4
Reading error samples	Shut = Shoot	
	Cleanse = Kleenex	
	Poise = Pose	
	Oxygen = Equation	
	Courage = Garage	
Pseudoword decoding error samples	Thag = Thang	
	Clait = Clant	
	Ruckid = Ricke	
Spelling error samples	Guess = Ges	
	Couldn't = Can't	
	Design = Deghin	
	Easier = Eser	

These data are classic examples of "pathognomonic signs" of Reading Disorder. First, two areas of language function that support reading ability are clearly impaired. Some practitioners might interpret scaled scores of 8, which are equivalent to the 25th %ile ranking, as falling within the low-average range; however, nothing could be further from the truth with respect to these Phonological Processing and Rapid Object Naming scores because *these skills do not follow a normal distribution. Performances on these tasks are highly skewed. Therefore, interpreting these skills as if they were high average, average, or low average does not do justice to the child who is attempting to demonstrate their abilities in these areas. The interpretations become diagnostically misleading and generate "false negative error."* The same is true of the Word Reading and Pseudoword Decoding subtests. Technically speaking, these scores undeniably fall within the low average range, and, one can argue that reading ability follows the normal distribution of a bell-shaped curve; *however, the characteristics of these reading errors demonstrate that this child does not understand the rules of reading because these mistakes do not follow phonemic/phonological principles. These mistakes illustrate that she is unable to integrate the phonological information that is conveyed by the letter sequences in these particular words.* Similarly, although no practitioner will deny that spelling ability at the 4th %ile ranking is indeed problematic, the "real" issue that emerges concerns her lack of appreciation of sound-symbol correspondences. Many practitioners may have been taught that the essence of neuropsychology is primarily its ability to quantify cognitive and behavioral samples. We have no argument with the usefulness of quantification of test information; however, as we have "perseverated" throughout this volume, the very definition of neuropsychology is the study of brain-behavior relationships. After test data have been scored, every interpretation is a series of "decision making points," as we have illustrated in the levels of inference we described in this manuscript. *The argument that quantitative interpretations are "better" than qualitative interpretations is a superficial argument in clinical evaluation. This is simply not the issue. Instead, we argue that by utilizing multiple levels of inferential interpretation, each "level" has a certain relative utility, but when these levels are combined, the real power of this clinical approach emerges as a synergistic diagnostic product.*

References

1. Reitan, R., & Wolfson, D. (2008). Can neuropsychological testing produce unequivocal evidence of brain damage? 1. Testing for specific deficits. *Applied Neuropsychology, 15*(1), 33–38.
2. Loring, D. W. (1999). *INS dictionary of neuropsychology* (p. 124). New York, NY: Oxford University Press.
3. Baron, I. S. (2004). *Neuropsychological evaluation of the child.* New York, NY: Oxford University Press.
4. Sbordone, R. J. (2001). Limitations of neuropsychological testing to predict the cognitive and behavioral functioning of persons with brain injury in real-world settings. *NeuroRehahilitation, 16*, 199–201.

5. Ashby, F. G., & Ennis, J. M. (2006). The role of the basal ganglia in category learning. In B. H. Ross (Ed.), *The psychology of learning and motivation* (Vol. 46, pp. 1–36). New York, NY: Elsevier.

6. Ashby, F. G., Ennis, J. M., & Spiering, B. J. (2007). A neurobiological theory of automaticity in perceptual categorization. *Psychological Review, 114*, 632–656.

7. Ashby, F. G., & O'Brien, J. B. (2005). Category learning and multiple memory systems. *Trends in Cognitive Sciences, 9*, 83–89.

8. Kaspar, J. C., & Sokolec, J. (1980). Relationship between neurological dysfunction and a test of speed of motor performance. *Journal of Clinical Neuropsychology, 2*, 13–21.

9. Reitan, R. M., & Wolfson, D. (2009). The Halstead-Reitan neuropsychological test battery for adults: Theoretical, methodological, and validation bases. In I. Grant & K. M. Adams (Eds.), *Neuropsychological assessment of neuropsychiatric and neuromedical disorders* (3rd ed., pp. 3–24). New York, NY: Oxford University Press.

10. Ito, M. (1997). Cerebellar microcomplexes. In J. D. Schmahmann (Ed.), *The cerebellum and cognition* (pp. 475–487). San Diego, CA: Academic Press.

11. Ito, M. (2011). *The cerebellum: Brain for an implicit self.* Upper Saddle River, NJ: FT Press.

12. Koziol, L. F., & Lutz, J. T. (2013). From movement to thought: The development of executive function. *Applied Neuropsychology: Child, 2*(2), 104–115.

13. Benton, A. L., Hamsher, K., Varney, N. R., & Spreen, O. (1983). *Contributions to neuropsychological assessment: A clinical manual.* New York, NY: Oxford University Press.

14. Yener, G. G., & Zaffos, A. (1999). Memory and the frontal lobes. In B. L. Miller & J. L. Cummings (Eds.), *The human frontal lobes: Functions and disorders* (pp. 288–303). New York, NY: Guilford Press.

15. Caplan, D. (2003). Aphasic syndromes. In K. M. Heilman & E. Valenstein (Eds.), *Clinical neuropsychology* (4th ed., pp. 14–34). New York, NY: Oxford University Press.

16. Bauer, R. M., & Demery, J. A. (2003). Agnosia. In K. M. Heilman & E. Valenstein (Eds.), *Clinical neuropsycholgy* (4th ed., pp. 236–295). New York, NY: Oxford University Press.

17. Salmon, D. P., & Bondi, M. W. (2009). Neuropsychological assessment of dementia. *Annual Review of Psychology, 60*, 257–282.

18. Poore, M. A., & Barlow, S. M. (2009). Suck predicts neuromotor integrity and developmental outcomes. *Perspectives on Speech Sciences and Orofacial Disorders, 19*, 44–51.

19. Nigg, J. T., Willcutt, E. G., Doyle, A. E., & Sonuga-Barke, E. J. (2005). Causal heterogeneity in attention-deficit/hyperactivity disorder: do we need neuropsychologically impaired subtypes? *Biological Psychiatry, 57*(11), 1224–1230.

20. Willcutt, E. G., Doyle, A. E., Nigg, J. T., Faraone, S. V., & Pennington, B. F. (2005). Validity of the executive function theory of attention-deficit/hyperactivity disorder: A meta-analytic review. *Biological Psychiatry, 57*(11), 1336–1346.

21. Greenberg, L. M. (2011). *The test of variables of attention (Version 8.0) [Computer software].* Los Alamitos, CA: The TOVA Company.

22. Riccio, C. A., Reynolds, C. R., Lowe, P., & Moore, J. J. (2002). The continuous performance test: A window on the neural substrates for attention? *Archives of Clinical Neuropsychology, 17*(3), 235–272.

23. Doyle, A. E., Biederman, J., Seidman, L. J., Weber, W., & Faraone, S. V. (2000). Diagnostic efficiency of neuropsychological test scores for discriminating boys with and without attention deficit-hyperactivity disorder. *Journal of Consulting and Clinical Psychology, 68*(3), 477–488.

24. Hinshaw, S. P., Carte, E. T., Sami, N., Treuting, J. J., & Zupan, B. A. (2002). Preadolescent girls with attention-deficit/hyperactivity disorder: II. Neuropsychological performance in relation to subtypes and individual classification. *Journal of Consulting and Clinical Psychology, 70*(5), 1099–1111.

25. Koziol, L. F., & Stevens, M. C. (2012). Neuropsychological assessment and the paradox of ADHD. *Applied Neuropsychology: Child, 1*(2), 79–89.

26. Koziol, L. F., Budding, D. E., & Chidekel, D. (2013). *ADHD as a model of brain-behavior relationships.* New York, NY: Springer.

27. Koziol, L. F. (2014). *The myth of executive functioning: Missing elements in conceptualization, evaluation, and assessment.* New York, NY: Springer.

28. Cohen, R. A. (2014). *Subcortical and limbic attentional influences. The neuropsychology of attention*. New York, NY: Springer.
29. Posner, M. I. (2004). *Cognitive neuroscience of attention*. New York, NY: Guilford Press.
30. Rosvold, H. E., Mirsky, A. F., Sarason, I., Bransome, E. D., Jr., & Beck, L. H. (1956). A continuous performance test of brain damage. *Journal of Consulting Psychology, 20*, 343–350.
31. Stevens, C., Lauinger, B., & Neville, H. (2009). Differences in the neural mechanisms of selective attention in children from different socioeconomic backgrounds: An event-related brain potential study. *Developmental Science, 12*(4), 634–646.
32. Yeo, B. T., Krienen, F. M., Sepulcre, J., Sabuncu, M. R., Lashkari, D., Hollinshead, M., … Buckner, R. L. (2011). The organization of the human cerebral cortex estimated by intrinsic functional connectivity. *Journal of Neurophysiolog, 106*(3), 1125–1165.
33. Castellanos, F. X., & Proal, E. (2012). Large-scale brain systems in ADHD: Beyond the prefrontal-striatal model. *Trends in Cognitive Sciences, 16*(1), 17–26.
34. Koziol, L. F., Joyce, A. W., & Wurglitz, G. (2014). The neuropsychology of attention: Revisiting the "Mirsky model". *Applied Neuropsychology: Child, 3*(4), 297–307.
35. Mirsky, A. F. (1987). Behavioral and psychophysiological markers of disordered attention. *Environmental Health Perspectives, 74*, 191–199.
36. Mirsky, A. F. (1996). Disorders of attention: A neuropsychological perspective. In G. R. Lyon & N. A. Krasnegor (Eds.), *Attention, memory, and executive function* (pp. 71–95). Baltimore, MD: Paul H. Brookes.
37. Mirsky, A. F., Anthony, B. J., Duncan, C. C., Ahearn, M. B., & Kellam, S. G. (1991). Analysis of the elements of attention: A neuropsychological approach. *Neuropsychology Review, 2*, 109–145.
38. Mirsky, A. F., & Duncan, C. C. (2004). The attention battery for children: A systematic approach to assessment. In G. Goldstein, S. R. Beers, & M. Hersen (Eds.), *Comprehensive handbook of psychological assessment* (pp. 277–292). Hoboken, NJ: Wiley.
39. Mirsky, A. F., Fantie, B., & Tatman, J. (1995). Assessment of attention across the lifespan. In R. L. Mapou & J. Spector (Eds.), *Neuropsychological assessment: A clinical approach* (pp. 17–48). New York, NY: Plenum.
40. Gordon, M. (1983). *The Gordon diagnostic system*. DeWitt, NY: Gordon Systems.
41. Robertson, I. H. (2004). Examining attentional rehabilitation. In M. I. Posner (Ed.), *Cognitive neuroscience of attention* (pp. 407–419). New York, NY: Guilford Press.
42. Hager, F., Volz, H. P., Gaser, C., Mentzel, H. J., Kaiser, W. A., & Sauer, H. (1998). Challenging the anterior attentional system with a continuous performance task: a functional magnetic resonance imaging approach. *European Archives of Psychiatry and Clinical Neuroscience, 248*, 161–170.
43. Schulz, K. P., Fan, J., Tang, C. Y., Newcorn, J. H., Buchsbaum, M. S., Cheung, A. M. & Halperin JM. (2004). Response inhibition in adolescents diagnosed with attention deficit hyperactivity disorder during childhood: an event-related FMRI study. *American Journal of Psychiatry, 161*, 1650–1657.
44. Stevens, M. C., Kiehl, K. A., Pearlson, G. D., & Calhoun, V. D. (2007). Functional neural networks underlying response inhibition in adolescents and adults. *Behavioural Brain Research, 181*(1), 12–22.
45. Wang, D., Buckner, R. L., & Liu, H. (2014). Functional specialization in the human brain estimated by intrinsic hemispheric interaction. *The Journal of Neuroscience, 34*(37), 12341–12352.
46. Koziol, L. F., Barker, L. A., & Jansons, L. (2015). Attention and other constructs: Evolution or revolution? *Applied Neuropsychology: Child, 4*(2), 123–131.
47. Denckla, M. B., & Reiss, A. L. (1997). Prefrontal-subcortical circuits in developmental disorders. In N. A. Krasnegor, G. R. Lyon, & P. S. Goldman-Rakic (Eds.), *Development of the prefrontal cortex: Evolution, neurobiology, and behavior* (pp. 283–294). Baltimore, MD: Paul H. Brookes.
48. Cortese, S., Kelly, C., Chabernaud, C., Proal, E., Di Martino, A., Milham, M. P., & Castellanos, F. X. (2012). Toward systems neuroscience of ADHD: A meta-analysis of 55 fMRI studies. *The American Journal of Psychiatry, 169*(10), 1038–1055.
49. Frank, M. J., Santamaria, A., O'Reilly, R. C., & Willcutt, E. (2007). Testing computational models of dopamine and noradrenaline dysfunction in attention deficit/hyperactivity disorder. *Neuropsychopharmacology, 32*, 1583–1599.

50. Frank, M. J., Scheres, A., & Sherman, S. J. (2007). Understanding decision-making deficits in neurological conditions: Insights from models of natural action selection. *Philosophical Transactions of the Royal Society of London, 362,* 1641–1654.
51. Douglas, V. I., Barr, R. G., Amin, K., O'Neill, M. E., & Britton, B. G. (1988). Dosage effects and individual responsivity to methylphenidate in attention deficit disorder. *Journal of Child Psychology and Psychiatry, 29*(4), 453–475.
52. Berridge, C. W., & Devilbiss, D. M. (2011). Psychostimulants as cognitive enhancers: the prefrontal cortex, catecholamines, and attention-deficit/hyperactivity disorder. *Biological Psychiatry, 69*(12), e101–111.
53. Wilens, T. E. (2008). Effects of methylphenidate on the catecholaminergic system in attention-deficit/hyperactivity disorder. *Journal of Clinical Psychopharmacology, 28*(3 Suppl 2), S46–S53.
54. Arnsten, A. F. T., & Pliszka, S. R. (2011). Catecholamine influences on prefrontal cortical function: relevance to treatment of attention deficit/hyperactivity disorder and related disorders. *Pharmacology, Biochemistry, and Behavior, 99*(2), 211–216.
55. Berridge, C. W., Devilbiss, D. M., Andrzejewski, M. E., Arnsten, A. F., Kelley, A. E., Schmeichel, B., … Spencer, R. C. (2006). Methylphenidate preferentially increases catecholamine neurotransmission within the prefrontal cortex at low doses that enhance cognitive function. *Biological Psychiatry, 60*(10), 1111–1120.
56. Rubia, K., Smith, A., Halari, R., Matukura, F., Mohammad, M., Taylor, E., & Brammer, M. J. (2009). Disorder-specific dissociation of orbitofrontal dysfunction in boys with pure Conduct disorder during reward and ventrolateral prefrontal dysfunction in boys with pure Attention-Deficit/Hyperactivity Disorder during sustained attention. *The American Journal of Psychiatry, 166,* 83–94.
57. Tana, M. G., Montin, E., Cerutti, S., & Bianchi, A. M. (2010). Exploring cortical attentional system by using fMRI during a continuous perfomance test. *Computational Intelligence and Neuroscience, 2010,* 329213. doi:10.1155/2010/329213.
58. Feifer, S. G., & Della Toffalo, D. A. (2007). *Integrating RTI with cognitive neuroscience: A scientific approach to reading.* Middletown, MD: School Neuropsych Press.
59. Shaywitz, S. (2003). *Overcoming dyslexia: A new and complete science-based program for reading problems at any level* (p. 123). New York, NY: Knopf.
60. Mann, V. (1998). Language problems: A key to early reading problems. In B. Wong (Ed.), *Learning about learning disabilities* (pp. 129–162). Orlando, FL: Academic Press.
61. Nicolson, R. (2000). Dyslexia and dyspraxia: Commentary. *Dyslexia, 6,* 203–204.
62. Nicolson, R. I., & Fawcett, A. (2005). Developmental dyslexia, learning and the cerebellum. In W. W. Fleischhacker & D. J. Brooks (Eds.), *Neurodevelopmental disorders* (pp. 19–36). Vienna, Austria: Springer.
63. Nicolson, R. I., & Fawcett, A. J. (2006). Do cerebellar deficits underlie phonological problems in dyslexia'? *Developmental Science, 9,* 259–262.
64. Nicolson, R. I., & Fawcett, A. J. (2007). Procedural learning difficulties: reuniting the developmental disorders'? *Trends in Neuroscience, 30,* 135–141.
65. Ackermann, H. (2008). Cerebellar contributions to speech production and speech perception: Psycholinguistic and neurobiological perspectives. *Trends in Neurosciences, 31*(6), 265–272.
66. Shaywitz, S. (1998). Current concepts: Dyslexia. *The New England Journal of Medicine, 338*(5), 307–312.
67. Koziol, L. F., Barker, L. A., & Jansons, L. (2015). Conceptualizing developmental language disorders: A theoretical framework including the role of the cerebellum in language-related functioning. In P. Marien & M. Manto (Eds.), *The linguistic cerebellum.* San Diego, CA: Academic Press.
68. Hillert, D. (2014). *The nature of language: Evolution, paradigms, and circuits.* New York, NY: Springer.
69. Mann, V. (1998). Language problems: A key to early reading problems. In B. Wong (Ed.), *Learning about learning disabilities* (pp. 213–228). Orlando, FL: Academic Press.
70. Miller, C. J., Sanchez, J., & Hynd, G. W. (2003). Neurological correlates of reading disabilities. In L. Swanson & S. Graham (Eds.), *Handbook of research on learning disabilities* (pp. 242–255). New York, NY: Guilford Press.

71. Bowers, P. G., & Ishaik, G. (2003). RAN's contribution to understanding reading disabilities. In S. Graham, H. Swanson, & K. R. Lee Harris (Eds.), *Handbook of learning disabilities* (pp. 140–157). New York, NY: Guilford Press.
72. Liberman, I. Y., Shankweiler, D., Fischer, F. W., & Carter, B. (1974). Explicit syllable and phoneme segmentation in the young child. *Journal of Experimental Child Psychology, 18,* 201–212.
73. Mann, V. A., & Liberman, I. Y. (1984). Phonological awareness and verbal short-term memory. *Journal of Learning Disabilities, 17,* 592–598.
74. Wolf, M. (1984). Naming, reading and the dyslexias: A longitudinal overview. *Annals of Dyslexia, 34,* 87–115.
75. Mann, V. A. (1984). Longitudinal prediction and prevention of early reading difficulty. *Annals of Dyslexia, 34*(1), 117–136.
76. Lezak, M. D., Howieson, D. B., Bigler, E. D., & Tranel, D. (2012). *Neuropsychological assessment* (5th ed.). New York, NY: Oxford University Press.

Chapter 6
Tradition and Innovation: Making the Neuropsychological Evaluation a More Powerful Tool

"Concentration: put all your eggs in one basket, and watch that basket."

Andrew Carnegie

"Become a possibilitarian. No matter how dark things seem to be or actually are, raise your sights and see possibilities- always see them, for they're always there."

Norman Vincent Peale

"Truth has no special time of its own. Its hour is now- always."

Albert Schweitzer

Most neuropsychological tests are blatantly explicit. By this, we mean that most of the tests we administer focus upon the concept and assumption of conscious cognitive control. In addition, many of these tasks appear to be artificial, and the results of these measures are difficult to correlate with day-to-day activities. For example, during the course of the day, people are not repeating digits forwards and backwards; they are not sorting cards into categories or solving "tower" tests; they are not connecting circles in numerical order with a pencil line, etc. Nevertheless, based upon interpretations of test results, we attempt to identify symptoms and diagnose pathology. The neuropsychologist then attempts to predict how the patient may present the in the "real world," making inferences from test interpretation. From this, the clinician attempts to devise meaningful interventions that will support the patient in treating and/or compensating for their deficiencies; however, many of the tasks that are administered in a neuropsychological battery are not practical, and thus performance on the measure may not translate or generalize well in terms of a patient's neurobehavioral presentation outside of the clinical setting. Some tests utilize game-like formats. Other tasks are administered conveying academic overtones, and still other tasks are administered within a question-answer format. So the inferences and predictions we make are always indirect.

© Springer International Publishing Switzerland 2016
L.F. Koziol et al., *Large-Scale Brain Systems and Neuropsychological Testing*,
DOI 10.1007/978-3-319-28222-0_6

A primary example of measures with academic overtones are the Wechsler scales, especially when a "group" of these tests is administered within a school setting; however, the Wechsler series has flaws with respect to the clinical utility of outcomes in a neuropsychological assessment. Although these "WIS" subtests were never originally intended to be used as neuropsychological instruments, this is not to say that the Wechsler series do not provide valuable information. And the Wechsler scales are perhaps the most "popular" tasks administered in neuropsychological testing [1]. Every set of tasks has limitations, and on nearly all WIS-like subtests, the examiner "guides" all of the activity. Similarly, these types of tasks are very explicit and based upon a static view of brain function [2]. And, as has been reviewed in *The Compendium of Neuropsychological Tests, 3rd Edition* [3], most examiners focus upon tests that are explicit, and the conclusion has been offered that considerable meaningful data is likely lost because of the lack of evaluating implicit procedures and processes.

A static view of brain function is inherent in current methodologies of neuropsychological assessment. *ADHD as a Model of Brain-Behavior Relationships* [49] and *The Myth of Executive Functioning* [50], this evaluation approach was referred to as the serial-order processing paradigm. This model is based upon the view that first, we perceive, second, we think in order to formulate a solution to a problem, and third, we finally act by implementing that solution. As reported by Cisek and Kalaska [4] and others [5, 6], there is very little evidence to support this type of serial order processing paradigm. It is certainly true that at times, we do engage in this type of problem-solving; however, this type of serial-order processing methodology does not account for or explain how smoothly, quickly, and effectively people are generally able to coordinate and control their adaptive behavior. This also might be thought of as a "perceive-think-respond" methodology that represents a variation of convergent thinking. In simplified terms, this means that problems are presented or that questions are asked, and that there really is only one way of solving the problem or correctly answering the question. This is clearly an explicit and almost completely an examiner-directed approach toward assessment; it is believed that as much as 95 % of behavior occurs on a routine, regular, automatic, and habitual basis. Therefore, much of thought and behavior must be implicit. Every day of our lives we do things that need to be done, without really thinking about them or how to do them. This is the essence of the novelty-routinization principle. In this regard, it is essential for the neuropsychologist to know how people learn implicitly. Similarly, problem-solving behavior that occurs "on-the-fly" would appear to require efficient perception/idea-action coupling that occurs quickly and implicitly [7]. These adaptive behaviors can be outside of our conscious awareness when they initially occur, though we are often able to recall them explicitly, later, after the "event" occurred. For example, think about driving on the expressway, thinking about something else as we drive, but then quickly stopping or turning to avoid an accident when something occurred that must have captured our attention.

The world of neuropsychology is changing. We can no longer think of behavior as organized along a verbal versus non-verbal dichotomy. We cannot view behavior in terms of verbal-visual-spatial functional differences. Instead, the neuroscientific evidence [8, 9] supports a novelty-routinization principle of vertebrate brain organization. As such, human brain-behavior relationships need to be viewed within that context. Any new task, by definition, is novel. Inherent in novelty is a change in the visual-spatial characteristics of that set of circumstances. Visual-spatial functioning can be viewed as nothing more than representing a change in the "momentary geometry" of any given, changing situation [10, 11]. When we are faced with a novel problem, we learn the solution to that problem, and if it is relevant and adaptive, a neuropsychologically intact individual will engage in that behavior over and over again, so that the behavior in question becomes automatic or routine. As we discussed in *ADHD as a Model of Brain-Behavior Relationships* [49] and *The Myth of Executive Functioning* [50], when this "automatic" or routine level of functioning is achieved, the behavior becomes independent of conscious cognitive control. Therefore, we might think of any novel behavior as initially requiring cognitive input or cognitive control in order to achieve a solution, but as that behavior is practiced or learned, it becomes independent of higher-order cognitive control [12]. This is the basic, fundamental principle that was described in the previously mentioned volumes as well.

Based upon this information, how can we make neuropsychological instruments that were developed and utilized years ago relevant to the significant advancements in our understanding of brain-behavior relationships and have these instruments align with what is known in the neurosciences? We now need to think in terms of the operations of the ventral and dorsal attention networks, the fronto-parietal network, the default mode network, the limbic network, and how all of these systems interact with the sensory and motor networks for the purpose of constantly interacting within a dynamically changing environment. We also need to think about how these networks operate in a segregated and in an integrated manner to support adaptive decision making. This is truly a daunting, formidable task. Furthermore, these networks interact with the gating mechanisms of the basal ganglia for the proper selection of behaviors [13–16], and they similarly interact with the cerebellar circuitry system in order to properly refine, automate, and adapt behavior as circumstances change. In fact, although we can understand certain test results and behaviors in terms of the cortico-basal ganglia gating mechanisms, such as the commission errors on a continuous performance test described in the previous chapter, practical clinical neuropsychology has no measures that assess the integrity of the cerebellum. Nevertheless, we believe that by altering certain methods of administration of currently available tests, we can just now begin to tap certain of these processes and functions. Similarly, perhaps we can revisit and revise certain traditional concepts in order to make them more applicable to current clinical neuropsychological practice.

Practice Effect: What Is It and Should It Always Be Avoided?

"Practice effect" refers to a general test-taking benefit in which test performance is enhanced after repeated administrations of the same test [17]. In fact, practice effects can also occur with different test items, because from one test administration to the next, the patient seems to learn how to approach a task more efficiently. In other words, the patient sometimes "learns" how to take the test. It has been suggested that practice effects are to be avoided, particularly because they interfere with the measurement of any given person's "true ability;" however, there is absolutely no universal agreement about whether or not "true ability" exists, nor is there agreement as to how this should be measured. People adjust to situations. This essentially means that the brain adjusts to situations. In fact, this is exactly what we expect a human brain to do. The brain takes a novel set of circumstances and it attempts to efficiently manage those circumstances by becoming more familiar with them, and by identifying methods of effective adaptation. The brain is continuously in a state of making what is unfamiliar or novel more familiar or even automatic to reduce the neurocognitive demands of the given behavior. This is how the human brain problem-solves. Even in normal control subjects, considerable test score variability is common from one test administration to another test administration even after relatively brief periods of time [18]. If our purpose is to study and understand brain-behavior relationships, then the concept of practice effect may not be a "bad thing" and, in fact, may be a valuable tool in terms of understanding an individual's neurocognitive status. Practice effects may, in fact, be a measure of the individual's learning efficiency or ability to take a novel process and make it automatic. We completely understand that this is our "novel," controversial opinion; we are asking neuropsychologists to stop and to think about the importance of what most practitioners were taught to avoid; at the same time, we are uncompromising in proposing that this viewpoint has relevance with respect to the study of brain-behavior relationships.

It is useful to break practice effect down into at least two different types. All cognitive tests consist of two basic elements, which comprise the broad categories of content and procedures [19]. All tasks simply must contain stimulus content, and most problem-solving tasks will also feature procedures. If these procedures are known, this will facilitate efficient solutions. Therefore, in some cases, it might be useful to separate practice effects into these two broad dimensions. In general, the neuroanatomic substrate for task *content* is the medial temporal lobe memory system, which requires the integrity of the hippocampus and related structures. This allows for the conscious recollection of the task, and more often than not, it is influenced by recognition recall and/or conscious awareness. The *learning and memory of procedures* recruits the cortico-basal ganglia system, often referred to under the "umbrella-like" category of the fronto-striatal system.

One task with both content and procedure that is extremely obvious is the Wisconsin Card Sorting Test (WCST). For example, the stimulus items consist of the shapes, colors, and the number of geometric forms. This is the explicit content. The procedural aspect concerns learning how to sort these cards along the proper dimensions in response to the informational "feedback" provided by the examiner as to whether the response is "correct" or "incorrect." If the task is re-administered on one or perhaps on several occasions, it is certainly true that the original intention of the task is no longer being measured, which is to "discover" the three organizing principles of color, form, and number; however, by comparing test performances after repeated administrations of the WCST, the neuropsychologist could effectively measure and assess if the patient learned the content and the procedure. Although this clearly changes the usual purpose or intent of the task, it also provides diagnostic information about the particular patient's ability to remember the content and learn the procedure. Although it is beyond the scope of this brief manuscript to discuss the purpose and administration of the WCST in greater detail, the fact that significant improvements are made across trials would be clinically relevant and of diagnostic import. In our view, overall view, the WCST is a problem-solving task that requires an individual to discover the stimulus-based properties that govern the problem in question. This viewpoint should not be surprising, because *The Myth of Executive Functioning* [50] was devoted to that topic; all problem solving requires an individual to discover the stimulus-based properties of the problem; however, if the task is re-administered without improvement in performance variables, this might indicate that the individual was unable to learn about the task characteristics. The ability or inability to learn the stimulus-based characteristics of the test would be of considerable clinical value. Presently there are no normative standards for making this type of judgment; therefore, this conclusion would need to be made with extreme caution.

The exact same overall principles would be applicable to other tasks, such as the traditional and well-known Block Design subtest. The stimulus-based characteristics are both observed in the content and the procedural elements of the task; the content concerns the different items which are essentially perceptions of the various configurations or patterns of the blocks; the procedural principles include the "discovery" that the 4 blocks make a square, and that this same "square" can be constructed without a framed outline; on 9-block items, the organizing principle changes to learning the underlying principle that all the solutions concern a 3×3 configuration, and that the stimulus "outline" can be removed, while even rotating the stimulus figures at a $90°$ angle, taking on a more abstract appearance. "Logical intuition" informs us that the understanding of these principles can be either explicit or implicit, although to our knowledge, this has never been formally investigated. In any event, *the concept of practice effect is based upon the idea that the individual is capable of benefiting from the experience of interacting within his or her environment. This is what the human brain is supposed to do as its primary functional goal!* With multiple administrations of the same task, we would expect that everyone's performance improves. Aspects of this type of learning can be implicit, which is seldom, if ever, measured through contemporary neuropsychological measures. Practice effects indicate that an individual has learned and can execute a set of procedures, without really having a conscious intention to do so when the task was initially administered. "Conscious awareness" might be necessary to initially discover these stimulus-based characteristics, but improved performance no longer requires the guidance of goal-directed thinking. We consider it essential that the field begin to develop and implement measures of procedural and implicit learning. However, the WCST and the Block Design subtest are relatively "easy," since the content of these tasks arguably out-weighs the "procedures." Nevertheless, people with certain pathologies might find these tests extremely difficult. It is sufficient to demonstrate that these tasks consist of both content and procedures, and that both explicit and implicit learning can be demonstrated through the effects of "practice," which is nothing more than repeated administration and performance.

The most widely known, classic case of medial temporal lobe anterograde amnesia is H.M. In 1953, in an effort to relieve severe epilepsy, he received a bilateral medial temporal lobe resection [20]. Since the time of his surgery, he was unable to learn and retain any new memories for events and information. However, as reviewed by Banich and Compton [21], H.M. was capable of learning new skills, such as the mirror tracing task, the rotary pursuit task, a mirror-reading task, and the Tower of Hanoi, a version of which is available on the DKEFS [22]. These tasks appear to be dependent upon perceptual-action coupling [23]. Although to our knowledge, it has never been conceptualized this way before, the dissociation between the declarative memory system and procedural learning system reveal the distinction between knowing "what" and knowing "how." And, we assess the medial temporal lobe system through a type of "practice effect," which is a way of thinking about the learning and memory assessed by administering the CVLT [24]. What neuropsychology is missing, and needs, is an evaluation of the learning and memory of the "how" system, in other words, the procedural learning system.

In our opinion, the original Trail Making Tests (TMT), which are in the public domain, represent an ideal candidate for evaluating an individual's ability to benefit from interacting with a task, traditionally known as practice effect; however, according to our proposed administration, we are evaluating implicit learning. This is the "how" system of procedural learning. Before introducing our methodology of administration, it is critical to examine the component brain systems that support successful task completion of the trail making tests. (The reader who is not familiar with the TMT should consult Strauss, et al., [3] and Lezak, et al., [1]).

The assumption that is made in order to complete TMT Part A is that the patient in question understands numerical sequence. It is also assumed that that the patient is able to recognize the numbers. The test consists of numbers within circles that are randomly distributed on a standard size sheet of paper. The test requires the patient to connect all of the numbers in proper ascending serial order with a pencil line as quickly as possible. The standard administration of this test consists of a single trial. The variable of interest concerns the speed with which the task is completed. If errors are made, this is pointed out to the subject for correction, and the errors negatively impact the patient's completion time.

Based upon current theoretical neuropsychological principles, we would expect this task to recruit the ventral attention network (VAN). The purpose of this brain region activation would be necessary for identifying the numbers. This is the case because the ventral attention network supports object identification, which is sometimes referred to as the "what" pathway [25]. In addition, it would be predicted that successful completion of this task activates the dorsal attention network (DAN). The dorsal attention network, consisting of connections between the frontal eye fields and the parietal lobes, would be activated for the purpose of locating the various numbers or, in other words, generating a meaningful visual-search strategy in order to locate the position of the numbers on the page. In this regard, aspects of the dorsal attention network have been referred to as the "where" pathway [25]. Holding the pencil in order to connect the numbers activates the sensory-motor network. Finally, in order to coordinate these operations, activation of the fronto-parietal network (FPN) would be expected as well. This would provide the appropriate cognitive control or guidance [26].

In our proposed administration, TMT Part A would be presented in five consecutive trials, rather than in a single trial based upon standard administration procedures. From the first trial to the last trial, we would expect improved performance as measured by a decrease in time to completion. Because the same stimulus page would be presented five times consecutively, all factors would remain constant. We would essentially be measuring the implicit learning of a novel, visual-search strategy which is dependent upon interactions between the VAN, DAN, and the FPN. The patient serves as his or her own normative control. During the course of completing this task over five trials, the prediction mechanisms of the cerebellum would be activated so that the hand would almost be guided by itself, motorically, becoming independent of conscious cognitive control and moving on the basis of "prediction." The cerebellum would learn the position of the numbers from prediction through repetition so that the final, best performance would be retained within the premotor cortex. Cerebro-cerebellar interactions would "learn" the implicit visual-search strategy, and the most efficient representation of that strategy, as measured by a decrease in time to completion, would be stored within the premotor cortex, because the cortex retains what the cerebellum learns [27]. This would represent the implicit learning function of the cerebellum, reflecting the brain's potential to develop automatic behaviors. This type of administration would be particularly useful and beneficial for patients who initially perform slowly, and/or with initial errors; however, if the subject immediately performs well within the range of normal limits with respect to speed and accuracy parameters on the initial, or perhaps even more quickly than expected, then the administration of five consecutive trials would not be necessary.

TMT Part B makes two assumptions. First, the same assumption is made that the individual in question knows the automated numeric sequence. The second assumption that is made relates to assuming that the individual has automated the alphabetic sequence. TMT Part B requires the individual to learn a new sequence by alternating between numbers and letters, letters to numbers, numbers to letters, and so on while maintaining ascending numeric and alphabetic ordering. The new sequence becomes 1-A-2-B-3-C-4-D and so on. This new sequence stops with the number 13 (on the adult version of the task). In the performance of this task, the same VAN, DAN, FPN, and SMN networks are presumably activated, for the same reasons as described above; however, TMT Part B introduces an additional requirement. From a global perspective, this additional requirement can perhaps describe the emphasis upon "working memory" functions; however, upon closer examination, in a neuroanatomic sense, there are more processes being recruited than just those thought to comprise working memory.

For example, the numeric sequence of 1-2-3-4-5 represents an extremely robust motor and well-established pattern. Similarly, the alphabetic sequence of A-B-C-D-E is just as robust. When we use the word "robust," we literally mean very strong and difficult to break. These types of cognitive/motor sequences are robust because they typically run their course. Once they start, they typically run through to their natural ending points, of course with the exception of numbers, which are infinite. Therefore, in the performance of TMT Part B, the "working memory" component actually consists of starting a robust sequence, breaking or interrupting the familiar sequence in favor of a novel sequence, and repeating this process over and over again until completion of the task. This is why summarizing this task as being one that is related to only working memory is inadequate. The initial breaking of the known sequences and integrating the new sequence is initially under cortical "conscious control" as frontal systems interact with the starting, stopping, and "chunking" processes of the basal ganglia ([28], see chapters 2, 4, 8, and 9). There is substantial mental tracking required while completing TMT Part B. While mental tracking is involved, our additional point concerns the breaking of the automated numeric and alphabetic sequences for the insertion of an aspect of another sequence, and then, breaking and combining aspects of both sequences on a continual basis in order to complete the task. In other words, we are describing a completely new perception-action coupling. The individual must interrupt a robust, automatic sequence constantly, while combining a perception with a new action. Since the cerebellum copies the content of working memory, in this case, the cortical-striatal interactions for the new sequence, and the locations of the numbers and letters, the cerebellum has the information it needs in order to "predict" and "automate." In our opinion, this is the essence of working memory—specifically, the coupling of a perception or idea with a new action. This is exactly how working memory functions guide behavior. Additionally, this is an extremely unique task because it is unlike other working memory testing tasks that are typically explicit. Once again, the uniqueness of this procedure concerns the perception-action coupling. This is the type of coupling that is necessary to engage in new behavior as we adjust to task novelty, while interacting within a dynamically changing environment.

It is true that the terms "shifting," "mentally tracking," and "working memory" can be terms that are used to describe TMT Part B; however, our emphasis upon this type of detail makes it considerably more clear as to what is actually required, which is consistent with our description of problem-solving processes that are described within the the previously mentioned volumes. In our administration protocol, we present TMT Part B over the course of five consecutive trials. Improved performance is measured by the elimination of errors and decreased time to task completion. By the time the fifth trial is administered, the normal control subject should be well on his or her way toward automating a new sequence of behavior (i.e., alternating an ascending numeric-alphabetic sequence). This represents a motor sequence that is actually cognitive in nature. When understood in this way, we argue that TMT Part B represents an extremely important tool for the practicing neuropsychologist, much more useful than it is right now in current administration practice, but only if we change administration standards by providing multiple, consecutive, and repetitive trials. Another way to administer this task would be to use as many trials as might be necessary to demonstrate task acquisition, indicating performance consistent with the majority of the individual's age-matched cohorts. However, the "5 trials" model controls for the number of stimulus presentations, while a "trials to acquisition" model might not be appropriate for all subjects while it introduces an additional variable which further complicates interpretation.

With respect to interpretation of the TMT task, a review of the normative standards provides little reason to believe that performance on TMT Part A and TMT Part B would be "normally distributed." We do not think there reason to believe that performance on these subtests follow a bell-shaped curve; however, regardless of this assumption, which has yet to be proven, we have already indicated that this task can be administered and interpreted according to an individual comparison standard. The goal is to ascertain how long it might take for any given individual to automate the novel sequence through the processes of implicit learning required in the completion of both TMT Part A and Part B; therefore, just as we have pointed out with respect to the measurement of anterograde amnesia, this type of implicit procedural learning process should be interpreted on an intra-individual comparison basis. It may be useful to know how an individual performs relative to a group standard on the initial trial of TMT Part A and Part B; however, in terms of implicit learning, the primary relevant variable concerns how the individual performs relative to himself or herself. When employing this methodology, the subject is literally acting as his or her own control. We also believe that administering the TMT over multiple trials provides considerably more information to the clinical examiner than a single administration trial could. In fact, while the term "processing speed" has always been elusive in terms of difficulties in finding a universally agreed upon definition, we believe that this type of perception-action coupling actually represents the essence of processing speed, making this term much easier to understand as a manifestation of executive, cognitive control in comparison to automaticity. Furthermore, this way of administering the TMT is completely consistent with the novelty-routinization principle. Multiple administrations of the TMT start with cognitive control and theoretically end with automaticity.

Case 7

This vignettes concerns a Caucasian female who was seen on two separate occasions. She presents with rather unique neurologic pathology. For example, her MRI findings include an absence of the cerebellar vermis, a fusion of the cerebellar hemispheres, and an absence of the primary fissure of the cerebellum. While these findings are compatible with romboencephalitis, the potential involvement of the trigeminal nerve suggests the possibility of an extremely rare disorder called Gomez-Lopez-Hernandez Syndrome, of which there are only 34 such cases on documented record [29]. MRI data also revealed fusion of the cerebellar tonsils, which extended 6 mm below the level of the foramen magnum, which met criteria for a diagnosis of Chiari I Malformation as well. Figure 6.1 illustrates the MRI findings. She was seen for neuropsychological evaluation on two separate occasions, initially at the age of 7 years old, and again when she was 11 years old. The data presented here are restricted to the TMT Parts A and B, Child Version.

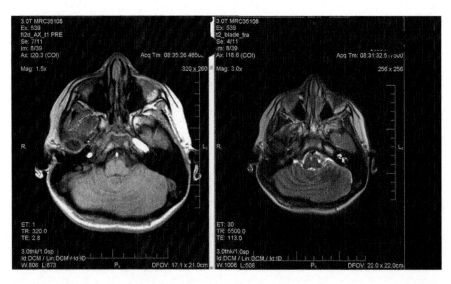

Fig. 6.1 MRI findings demonstrating a fusion of the cerebellar hemispheres, the absence of the primary fissure of the cerebellum, and agenesis of the cerebellar vermis. There is also a fusion of the cerebellar tonsils. The patient's presentation was confirmed as the 35th case on record with a diagnosis of Gomez-Lopez-Hernandez Syndrome

Test results		
7 years old		
Trail making test	Time	Errors
Trial A1	40″	2
Trial A2	22″	1
Trial A3	20″	0
Trial A4	19″	1
Trial A5	26″	0
Trial B1	66″	0
Trial B2	37″	0
Trial B3	66″	0
Trial B4	29″	0
Trial B5	71″	0

Test results		
11 years old		
Trail making test	Time	Errors
Trial A1	21″	0
Trial A2	13″	0
Trial A3	11″	0
Trial A4	12″	0
Trial A5	11″	1

Test results		
11 years old		
Trial B1	24″	0
Trial B2	21″	1
Trial B3	16″	1
Trial B4	14″	0
Trial B5	29″	3

These case data sets were not presented because of the rarity of the disorder. Instead, it needs to be kept in mind that the "easy" child version of TMT was administered on both occasions. This individual's general level of intellectual functioning was never a question, so that in order to satisfy anyone's curiosity about possible "cognitive referencing," global cognitive capacity has always been well within the range of expected, normal limits; however, at the age of seven, this child's performance did not give evidence that she was able to automate the very simple version of TMT Part A. On TMT Part B, though her performance was error-free, her functioning with respect to speed parameters was indicative of a lack of automaticity of the visual-search strategy. Scores ranged from average to two- and three-standard deviations below the mean, with unpredictable speed of performance from one trial to the next trial.

When she was seen at again at 11 years old, she performed much more quickly on TMT Part A, as might be expected, given her age at that time; however, it is difficult to argue whether the visual field search strategy was automated in light of the fact that, on the final trial, a very simple counting error was made. On TMT Part B, although speed of performance might be considered well within the range of expected limits, she made errors, and the mistakes she made were unpredictable from one trial to the next trial. This child made different mistakes each time she committed an error; therefore, once again, there was no persuasive evidence that this child was able to learn a visual search strategy. In our opinion, these data represent dramatic evidence of a lack of automatize, especially in view of the fact that serial test results were obtained, separated by a time frame of almost exactly 4 years. However, even without knowing about the cerebellar abnormalities within this individual's presentation, this type of performance can be observed in any patient that might walk into any clinician's office, on any given day. This young lady's neurocognitive profile reveals a certain level of cognitive control, although this was unreliable as evidenced in her committing errors. When reviewing the speed of her performance one may infer that the "DAN network" was unable to assist in automating the behavior. This is suggested by the fact that the cortex and cerebellum function as an ensemble, while vermal and lateral cerebellar regions would support performance. By definition, her condition includes difficulties in controlling reflexive eye movements; this does not invalidate the data but instead, it emphasizes the role of the FEF within the DAN. Therefore, this presentation illustrates the potential value of consecutive administrations of the TMT, which, in fact, is the only point we wish to make.

Perception/Idea-Action Coupling

What is perception-action coupling? At base, we are referring to perception-action coupling as an element of "working memory." In *The Myth of Executive Functioning* [50], it was described how working memory cannot possibly be a unitary entity, while it was also characterized as a process that is comprised of both explicit and implicit components that interact [30]. Perception-action coupling is similarly a multiple-component process [31, 32]. For example, many clinical tests that require the subject to copy geometric forms/designs are described as *"visual-motor"* tests. An aspect of executive functioning, in this case "working memory," implicitly lies in the "dash" between these two words [33]. The Rey Complex Figure Test [34] is a "visual-motor test" that requires the self-generation of organization. In order to draw the figure properly (and obtain the required 34–35 raw score points), the subject must ask himself/herself, either explicitly or implicitly, "how" to best draw the stimulus figure. This determination or manipulation of perceptions and/or ideas "occurs" within working memory. And these are the explicit, or implicit ideas that "guide" the drawing of the figure. And this literally *is* perception-action coupling, an aspect of working memory. The term "visual-motor" tells us nothing at all specific; but considering the term "visual-motor" within the framework of perception-action coupling, we are beginning to understand any given subject's "executive functioning" in the performance of this copying task.

The Rey-Osterreith Complex Figure Test, now usually referred to as the Rey Complex Figure Test (RCFT), which was once within the public domain, can therefore be utilized and interpreted as a measure that demonstrates how thought guides action. We have adopted a modified version of the RCFT test administration to demonstrate the process of perception-action coupling. Through this process, we have noticed that, even for normal control subjects, the "immediate memory" condition of this test tolerates or allows for considerable error. For example, normal control subjects can generate a reasonably accurate "copy" of the figure, earning a raw score between 35 and 36 points; however, just a few minutes later when the individual is asked to draw the complex figure from memory, a raw score of approximately 23–24 remains a satisfactory test performance. Therefore, even normal control subjects are seemingly allowed to "forget" considerable information in their reproductions and still obtain scores that would be considered representative of adequate recall. This most likely occurs because the subject has one limited exposure when copying the figure, and the "immediate memory" trial, which is not "immediate" at all because it occurs 3 min after the figure was copied, is an *incidental learning and recall task*, highly dependent upon how the subject initially organized and paid attention to what they were doing as they drew the figure. All practitioners who use this test must have noticed that subjects frequently approach the copy phase in a disorganized manner. Poor planning increases the likelihood of a poor copying score, and increases the likelihood of significant "forgetting" on the immediate memory and delayed recall conditions. More often than not, these types of performances are labeled as "visual-spatial" deficits; however, in our opinion, nothing could be further from the truth. Again, the manner in which the RCFT is administered is really an incidental learning task. The raw score data may imply that normal control subjects did not necessarily "pay attention" to what they are doing when copying the figure. When a disorganized approach towards copying is observed, how can anyone expect the individual to demonstrate an acceptable performance after just a few minutes, let alone in a lengthier delay condition? In this case, a false positive error would have been committed if one diagnosed "visual-spatial" deficits based upon a poorly planned and organized approach to the copy portion which resulted in poor encoding and retrieval of information.

In our view, difficulties in copying the RCFT may result from problems in perception-action coupling, when the subject does not ask himself/herself the relevant questions, either explicitly in consciousness or implicitly, about how to efficiently copy the figure. Therefore, when a disorganized approach at copying is observed, and after we complete the administration of the test in the standardized way, we proceed with a modified method of administration. This consists of the examiner drawing the figure for the subject. The figure is drawn in an organized way, and the examiner names every element for the subject, through active demonstration as the subject observes the copying. For example, as we draw the figure, we initially point out that perhaps the most obvious feature concerns the rectangle. We then proceed over to the right side of the page, and indicate that the portion of the figure on the right seems to resemble a triangle. We then proceed to draw the details of the figure, starting with the largest details and working to the smallest details. We draw the vertical line and the horizontal line, and we label these lines as such. We count the number of lines in the upper left hand quadrant and we draw that. We then count the number of lines that bifurcate the lower right corner diagonal, and we proceed to draw them as we name them. As we move to the upper right hand quadrant, we draw the circle with three dots, informing the subject that sometimes people might refer to this as a face, while at other times, some people refer to this as what might look like a bowling ball. We proceed to draw the figure in an organized fashion, labeling every element, until the figure is complete.

After this demonstration, we ask the subject to draw the figure in the exact same way that we drew it. We ask them to copy the figure again, and to silently talk themselves through the drawing process while silently labeling each aspect of the design. When the subject completes the drawing in this organized fashion, we then ask which way of drawing the figure was easier: the patient's original way, or the more organized approach demonstrated by the examiner. Most patients agree that they preferred the examiner's method for organizing the drawing. Then, we distract the patients by engaging in another task for approximately 3 min. We then present the subject with a blank sheet of paper, and we ask the subject to recall as much of the figure as possible. In this phase of the test administration, we almost always obtain a significantly improved drawing. We then present the patient with a blank sheet of paper approximately 3 min later, and we ask them to draw the figure again. We observe that nearly all patients are,

again, capable of reproducing a dramatically improved design. We then administer a 30 min recall. In fact, some of the authors of this manuscript have asked the
patients for a 24-h recall when the patient is seen on two consecutive days. Once
again, we find that most of the figure is retained. So in this modified administration methodology, the patient generates five sample "products": standard copy
administration and immediate recall; this is followed by another copy phase after
the patient observes a systematic drawing of the figure, followed again by immediate and delayed recall trials, all for purposes of comparison. A sixth recall after
24 h is optional, dependent upon circumstances. These multiple trials are all
interpreted according to an individual comparison standard, so that the subject
acts as his/her own control or "baseline."

By administering the task in this modified way, several important points are
clarified. First, the "traditional," and often "knee-jerk" interpretation of "visual-
spatial deficit" is immediately taken off the table. An improved performance
after using the "demonstration methodology" illustrates the person can draw,
that the subject paid attention to what they were doing, and that he/she "retained"
a good approximation of the stimulus figure. This must mean the VAN and DAN
were recruited for perception and analysis, and that the FPN and SMN were
recruited for successful execution of the task. A lack of integrity within these
systems, if properly identified and interpreted, would not be transient in the vast
majority of cases; instead, a stable but poor level of functioning in these areas
would be predicted. Second, the individual demonstrated that memory for that
type of material is intact. If this interpretation was incorrect, whether or not
every aspect of the design was labeled, poor information retrieval would be
expected, evidenced by poor performance in spite of the demonstrated, planned
approach. Therefore, in this modified administration, false positive error can
often be reduced or even eliminated. Interpretatively useful information is easily obtained. Furthermore, the integrity of perception-action coupling, the critical "linkage system" within working memory, is demonstrated by inference. To
prove these points, the individual's cognitive control system is initially supported by the examiner. Through the utilization of this process of administration, the examiner supports the examinee in coupling a perception with the
appropriate action. Once that linkage is established, the patient is able to function at a level consistent with the majority of normal control subjects. The individual learns how to guide action, or behavior. In delayed recall conditions, this
methodology also mimics how the subject recruits the Default Mode Network
(DMN), for drawing upon prior experiences to guide current "actions," or
behaviors.

Case 8

This is a case vignette of a 14 year old female who was seen for an evaluation of
ADHD. The copy phase of the RCFT was reasonably accurate, but when observing her
performance, the approach to drawing the figure seemed poorly organized. She first

drew the upper left external detail; this was followed by the horizontal line on the bottom of the figure; next came the "box" in the lower left aspect of the design and the horizontal line from it; this was followed by the top horizontal line, and then the vertical line extending throughout the figure and connecting to the horizontal line that runs from the lower left corner "box." All of the quadrants were drawn as independent segments—this can easily be determined by inspecting the final product, since the horizontal, vertical, and diagonal lines do not properly intersect, usually a tell-tail sign of a disorganized drawing approach. From our observational experience, we have concluded that unless an individual draws the outline initially, which provides a Gestalt framework, it is very difficult to recall the figure, even upon "immediate recall," without even providing a 3-min interval before recall. However, just as Shorr and colleagues found in neuropsychiatric populations, fragmentary recall, and/or aspects of "configurations" or perceptual clustering on recall trials is a significantly better predictor of memory performance than is initial copy accuracy [35]. This proved to be the case for this patient's recall. The figures for "CASE II" illustrate this, as well as the fact that this individual was able to benefit from the "demonstration approach," which improved the copying of the figure, while dramatically demonstrating notably improved recall, both after 3 min and after 24 h. These data provide a classic example of how the "textbook" administration would have inevitably generated a false positive error, not to mention the omission of the substantive information that was gained by modifying the administration. This clinical information includes the fact this adolescent demonstrated disorganization when completing a novel, problem-solving drawing task independently, that she was capable of "learning" the "working memory" and perception-action coupling necessary for task completion, while suggesting she would benefit from structured, directed treatment and management approaches.

- Slide 2=Patient's copy – standard administration with disorganized approach to drawing the figure
- Slide 3=Patient's Immediate recall after standard administration of copy
- Slide 4=Patient's copy after demonstration
- Slide 5=Patient's Immediate recall after demonstrating how to draw figure
- Slide 6=Patient's recall after 24 hours

In this regard, we are well aware of the controversy concerning the evidence to support the use of the RCFT in the measurement of executive functioning in children [36]. However, many studies use children from young school age through adolescence in their samples, and we cannot expect such a broad age-range to execute the task with the same level of skill sets [37]. Studies also correlate RCFT performance with other measures of executive function task performance and find weak relationships, but this

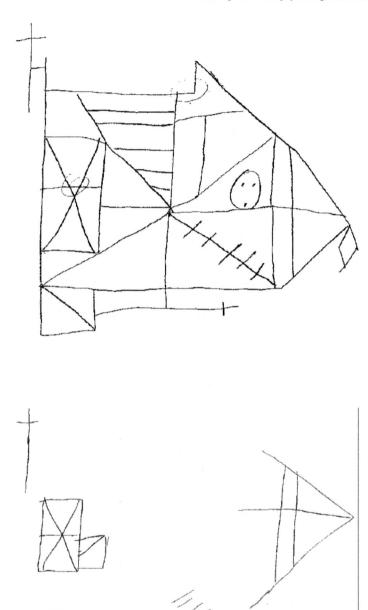

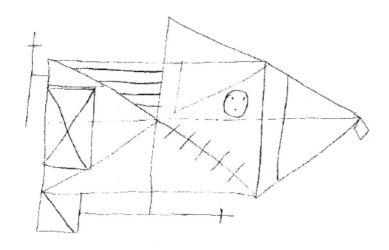

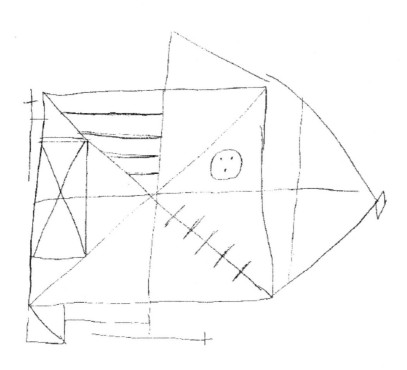

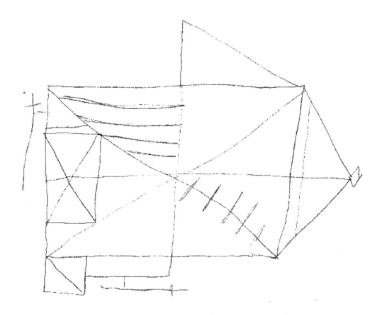

should be expected. In our view, and as presented in *ADHD as a Model of Brain-Behavior Relationships* [49] and *The Myth of Executive Functioning* [50], executive functions are not a monolithic entity. Cole [38] found that tasks always recruit multiple and different brain regions, and we posit that there is no "executive function" per se, but instead, FPNs that flexibly recruit whatever brain regions are required to complete any given task. This consists of a dynamically changing functional neuroanatomic substrate that is always task dependent. In this way, executive functioning can never be defined or understood apart from the task which is used to assess it. And, to the extent that the RCFT requires perception-action linkages, either explicitly or implicitly, it is dependent upon a process of working memory, in which perceptions/ideas guide action, or test performance. And, this requires a paradigm shift in the way in which we understand terms such as "executive function" and "working memory."

Case 9: RCFT Evidence of Compromised Functioning Within the VAN, DAN, FPN, AND SMN Systems

This is a case presentation of a 13 year old girl with poorly functioning brain systems, most likely within the VAN, DAN, FPN, and SMN systems. These inferences are derived on the basis of her RCFT drawings Based upon this deficit, we would predict deficits in novel problem-solving. She obtained an average range score on the VCI; this is in very sharp contrast to her other composite index scores which typically are not as useful or revealing as they are in her case. She obtained impaired-range scores, all between the second and fifth percentile rankings, on the PRI, WMI, and PSI WISC-IV indices. This child's history includes attention and executive function deficiencies, mixed dyslexia, dyscalculia, dysgraphia, and developmental coordination disorder. She presented with a "mixed bag" of clinical findings. She behaved in a socially out-of-step manner, but was not diagnosed with autism. Her behavior was often petulant and she failed to see her role in the negative outcomes of her decision making. This is an absolutely "perfect" presentation from which the clinical practitioner can gain important insights for understanding her adaptive difficulties.

The patient earned a <0.02 percentile rank on the RCFT Copy task. Her approach to the task was very disorganized. For example, she started by drawing the circle with three dots. The examiner then taught the child how to copy the drawing. Her performance improved from five correct items to 15, which only yielded a 0.04 percentile. Information she encoded was available for recall on the 30-min delayed recall trial (0.3 percentile). This performance shows how the child did not appreciably benefit from teaching, but that information she encoded was available for recall. The net outcome of this RCFT clearly points to the suspicion of a lack of integrity within the brain systems presumably measured, even though the examiner deviated from the above described modified administration, which omitted the patient's first immediate recall sample. But why are these behavioral samples still important?

Rey O Copy

Rey O Teaching

Rey O 3 Min

Rey O 30 Min

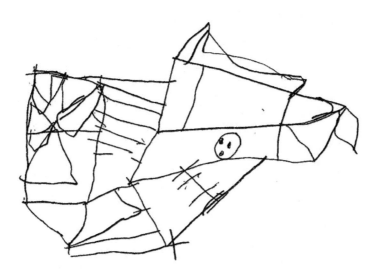

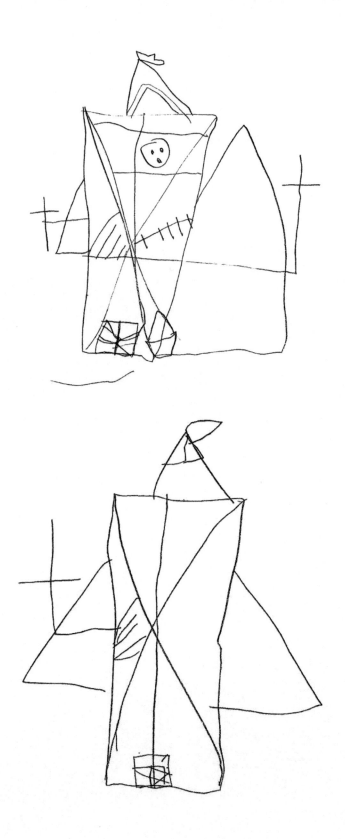

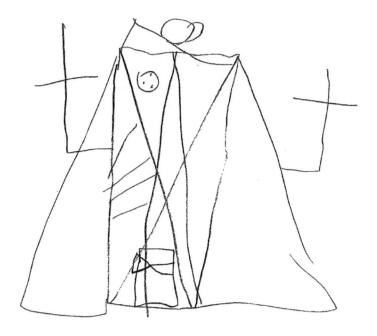

There are three specific reasons, all of equal importance. First, as described in *The Myth of Executive Functioning* [50], the right hemisphere can be considered a novelty detector. It is critical for problem-solving, which, by definition, is novel. In ambiguous, novel situations, the human brain makes choices and decisions not only by applying information learned from prior experiences (the DMN), but instead, adaptive behaviors are also defined by the momentary "geometry" of the immediate environment and change during continuously ongoing activity, or dynamically changing interactions [39]. Second, the right hemisphere is not irrelevant to language. Input from this hemisphere is clearly necessary for processing linguistic information such as the resolution of ambiguity when words have multiple meanings, metaphorical understanding, appreciation of humor, judgment and expression of affective language prosody, as well as the processing of the figurative and pragmatic aspects of language; all of these linguistic properties are driven by external factors that change dynamically as an inherent property of ongoing conversational discourse [9, 40]. Third, Vakalopoulos presented a very comprehensive, detailed, compelling neurodevelopmental review about how "visual-motor" ability and motor skills contribute to empathic dysfunction, again affecting social, interactive behaviors [41]. So once again, as was emphasized in the previously mentioned volumes [49, 50], it is not at all feasible to isolate "visual-spatial" skills as relegated to some sort of artificial compartment, and therefore relatively unimportant because we live in a "verbal world." Any fixed hemispheric assignment as in the "traditional" verbal versus visual-spatial dichotomy is unequivocally false, overly simplistic, and diagnostically misleading. Regardless of what any practitioner may have been taught, we need two functional, interacting cerebral hemispheres in order to achieve practical, successful adjustment. There is absolutely no evidence with which to generate a contrary neuroscientific viewpoint.

Therefore, the practitioner can readily extrapolate this information to her "real life" circumstances, without "bending," or "stretching," one single aspect of the data, while "reviewing" the neurobiologic substrates of her presentation with information derived from what we know about large scale brain systems. Although reading is first and foremost a language based skill, perceptual skills are also an early basic underpinning, although presently most likely in a minimal way as demonstrated through numerous investigations reviewed by Mann [42, 43]. Mathematics recruits a wide variety of skills, and a range of functional connectivity patterns between brain networks to support them, in order to execute computation problems and engage in borrowing, carrying, and division, etc. [44–46]. The neuroanatomic underpinnings can also be extrapolated, or inferred, from Voogd and colleagues [47], who identified the comprehensive, detailed neuroanatomy of "visual-motor" behavior. This child was also notably clumsy, which also reflects deficits in spatial-motor functioning. The neuroanatomic underpinning involves integrating information from the VAN and DAN with the sensori-motor network, or SMN ([26, 48]; Please see *ADHD as a Model of Brain-Behavior Relationships* [49] and *The Myth of Executive Functioning* [50], for additional information to provide the appropriate framework.) In short, by understanding the requirements of existing neuropsychological tests, and by possessing a working knowledge of large scale brain systems, considerable information can be derived about a subject's presentation, as well as practically useful, predictive information about the likely course of outcome, all of which can assist in dictating treatment planning and implementation (Unfortunately, additional intervention data are beyond the scope of this chapter).

Case 10: "Everything that Counts Cannot Be Counted"

This 10 year old boy was evaluated for Attention Deficit Hyperactivity Disorder. The examiner deviated from the modified administration procedure described above. First, the standard copy version was administered, followed by the boy's copying the figure again, followed by 3 and 30 min recall administrations. These drawings are depicted below. Upon initial administration, the patient's product was decent upon visual inspection, but in observing him draw, his approach was markedly disorganized. After he observed a systematic drawing of the RCFT, a subtle but significant improvement in his drawing was observed, and his copying approach was considerably improved. His immediate and delayed recall of the RCFT were both intact, although admittedly, a baseline of an initial immediate recall was not available for comparison purposes.

This case presentation remains important because the direction in which patients deploy or allocate attention while copying a figure informs the examiner about how the person analyzes and solves "spatial" problems. In other words, novel problem solving approaches are often revealed. To a large extent, we are all dependent upon the visual system. This should already be obvious, since the visual network (VN) supports the functions of both the VAN and DAN, as well as providing support for brain systems to inhibit responding to distracting influences ([26]; see the previously mentioned volumes for additional discussion). Even a seemingly common, basic task such as using a pencil and paper can provide the examiner with useful information about any given individual's integrity of brain systems functioning [19].

Order of Pictures:
1: Rey-O Copy
2: Rey-O Teaching
3: Rey-O 3 Minute Recall
4: Rey-O 30 Minute Recall

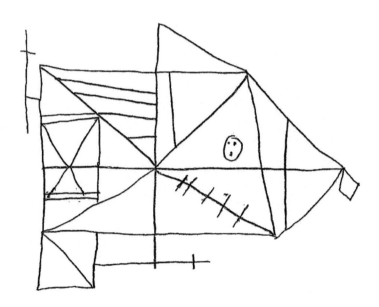

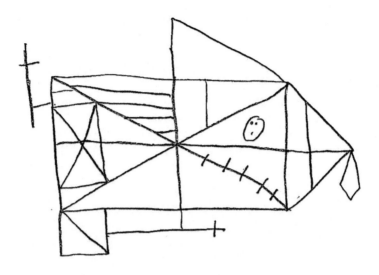

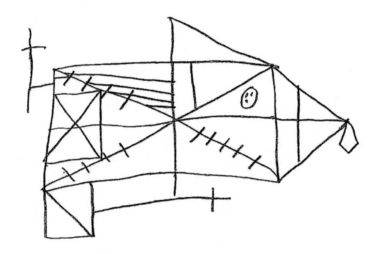

Summary

In the above examples we have demonstrated that inefficient or ineffective executive functioning/cognitive control can be mediated through structure, observation, and the cognitive guidance of an examiner. We demonstrated that patients were able to learn from the experience of interacting with both the examiner and the

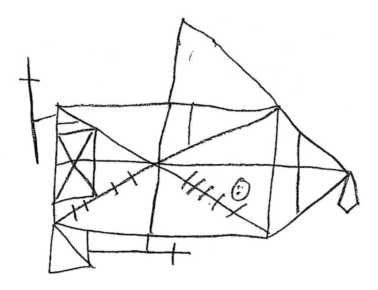

activity in which they were engaged. We also demonstrated that explicit learning processes may translate to implicit memory processes. The RCFT cases illustrated how the process of demonstration can be useful in "pinpointing" areas of deficit, and in predicting possibly expected behaviors and general principles about structuring treatment/management. Therefore, during this administration, we acquired considerably more information about the patients than we would have by simply relying upon a standardized administration methodology. Finally, within this type of administration, the performance of a normal control subject has nothing to do with the outcome we attempted to demonstrate. Instead, we were able to use the patient as his or her own control, and then utilize an individual comparison standard in order to obtain clinically useful conclusions. We reviewed how it is possible to avoid false positive errors.

Overall, this chapter revealed how commonly available neuropsychological tests can be made more clinically useful. By going against the status quo which we believe assesses cognition from a static viewpoint, we modified current test administration practices in order to evaluate a person's neuropsychological status from a dynamic perspective. We proposed a paradigm for assessing the individual's ability to adapt and automate behaviors. We firmly believe that the primary purpose of thinking is to guide interactive behavior within a dynamically changing environment. This requires perception/idea—action coupling, an element of "working memory," and we demonstrated that the Trail Making Tests and the RCFT can be administered and interpreted in an attempt to evaluate different aspects of this type of linkage. The next step in this process should be comprised of two critical components. First, systematic investigations need to be geared towards obtaining data from large groups of subjects in order to determine if our hypotheses are correct.

Second, these studies need to be correlated not with other neuropsychological tests, but instead, with controlled observations, through the development of appropriate questionnaires, in order to determine whether or not what we have measured really is associated with practical, daily behaviors such as routines, as well as minor changes in these routines to determine if these paradigms are ecologically valid.

References

1. Lezak, M. D., Howieson, D. B., Bigler, E. D., & Tranel, D. (2012). *Neuropsychological assessment* (5th ed.). New York, NY: Oxford University Press.
2. Hassin, R. R., et al. (2009). Implicit working memory. *Consciousness and Cognition, 18*(3), 665–678.
3. Strauss, E., Sherman, E. M. S., Spreen, O., & Spreen, O. (2006). *A compendium of neuropsychological tests: Administration, norms, and commentary.* Oxford, England: Oxford University Press.
4. Cisek, P., & Kalaska, J. F. (2010). Neural mechanisms for interacting with a world full of action choices. *Annual Review of Neuroscience, 33,* 269–298.
5. Singer, W. (2001). Consciousness and the binding problem. *The Annals of the New York Academy of Sciences, 929,* 123–146.
6. Shadlen, M. N., & Movshon, J. A. (1999). Synchrony unbound: A critical evaluation of the temporal binding hypothesis. *Neuron, 24*(1), 67–77. 111–125.
7. Bertenthal, B. I. (1996). Origins and early development of perception, action, and representation. *Annual Review of Psychology, 47,* 431–459.
8. Koziol, L. F., Barker, L. A., & Jansons, L. (2015). Attention and other constructs: Evolution or revolution? *Applied Neuropsychology: Child, 4*(2), 123–131.
9. Koziol, L. F., Barker, L. A., & Jansons, L. (2015). Conceptualizing developmental language disorders: A theoretical framework including the role of the cerebellum in language-related functioning. In P. Marien & M. Manto (Eds.), *The linguistic cerebellum.* San Diego, CA: Academic.
10. Cisek, P., & Kalaska, J. F. (2005). Neural correlates of reaching decisions in dorsal premotor cortex: Specification of multiple direction choices and final selection of action. *Neuron, 45,* 801–814.
11. Koziol, L. F., Barker, L. A., Hrin, S., & Joyce, A. W. (2014). Large-scale brain systems and subcortical relationships: Practical applications. *Applied Neuropsychology: Child, 3*(4), 264–273.
12. Ito, M. (2011). *The cerebellum: Brain for an implicit self.* Upper Saddle River, NJ: FT Press.
13. Redgrave, P., Prescott, T. J., & Gurney, K. (1999). The basal ganglia: A vertebrate solution to the selection problem? *Neuroscience, 89*(4), 1009–1023.
14. Cockburn, J., & Frank, M. J. (2011). Reinforcement learning, conflict monitoring, and cognitive control: An integrative model of cingulate-striatal interactions and the ERN. In R. B. Mars, J. Sallet, M. F. S. Rushworth, & N. Yeung (Eds.), *Neural basis of motivational and cognitive control.* Cambridge, MA: MIT Press.
15. Miller, R. (2008). *A theory of basal ganglia and their disorders.* Boca Raton, FL: CRC Press.
16. Doll, B., & Frank, M. J. (2009). The basal ganglia in reward and decision making: computational models and empirical studies. In J.-C. Dreher & L. Tremblay (Eds.), *Handbook of reward and decision making* (pp. 399–425). Oxford: Academic Press.
17. McCaffrey, R. J., Duff, K., & Westervelt, H. J. (2000). *Practitioner's guide to evaluating change with neuropsychological assessment instruments.* New York, NY: Kluwer Academic/Plenum.
18. Watkins, M. W., & Smith, L. G. (2013). Long-term stability of the Wechsler Intelligence Scale for Children—Fourth Edition. *Psychological Assessment, 25*(2), 477–483.
19. Milberg, W. P., Hebben, N., & Kaplan, E. (1996). The Boston process approach to neuropsychological assessment. In I. Grant & K. M. Adams (Eds.), *Neuropsychological assessment of neuropsychiatric disorders* (pp. 58–80). New York, NY: Oxford University Press.

20. Squire, L. R., & Shimamura, A. P. (1996). The neuropsychology of memory dysfunction and its assessment. In I. Grant & K. Adams (Eds.), *Neuropsychological assessment of neuropsychiatric disorders* (pp. 232–262). New York, NY: Oxford University Press.
21. Banich, M. T., & Compton, R. J. (2011). *Cognitive neuroscience* (3rd ed.). Belmont, CA: Wadsworth, Cengage Learning.
22. Delis, D. C., Kaplan, E., & Kramer, J. H. (2001). *Delis-Kaplan executive function system (D-KEFS)*. San Antonio, TX: The Psychological Corporation.
23. Saint-Cyr, J. A., & Taylor, A. E. (1992). The mobilization of procedural learning: The "key signature" of the basal ganglia. In L. R. Squire & N. Butters (Eds.), *The neuropsychology of memory* (2nd ed., pp. 188–202). New York, NY: Guilford Press.
24. Delis, D. C., Kramer, J. H., Kaplan, E., & Ober, B. A. (2000). *California verbal learning test* (2nd ed.). San Antonio, TX: Psychological Corporation.
25. Blumenfeld, H. (2010). *Neuroanatomy through clinical cases* (2nd ed.). Sunderland, MA: Sinauer.
26. Castellanos, F. X., & Proal, E. (2012). Large-scale brain systems in ADHD: Beyond the prefrontal-striatal model. *Trends in Cognitive Sciences, 16*(1), 17–26.
27. Galea, J. M., Vazquez, A., Pasricha, N., de Xivry, J. J., & Celnik, P. (2011). Dissociating the roles of the cerebellum and motor cortex during adaptive learning: The motor cortex retains what the cerebellum learns. *Cerebral Cortex, 21*, 1761–1770.
28. Koziol, L. F., & Budding, D. E. (2009). *Subcortical structures and cognition: Implications for neuropsychological assessment*. New York, NY: Springer.
29. de Mattos, V. F., Graziadio, C., Machado Rosa, R. F., Lenhardt, R., Alves, R. P., Trevisan, P., … Zen, P. R. (2014). Gómez-López-Hernández syndrome in a child born to consanguineous parents: new evidence for an autosomal-recessive pattern of inheritance? *Pediatric Neurology, 50*(6), 612–615.
30. Ansorge, U., Kunde, W., & Kiefer, M. (2014). Unconscious vision and executive control: How unconscious processing and conscious action control interact. *Consciousness and Cognition, 67*, 268–287.
31. Méndez, J. C., Pérez, O., Prado, L., & Merchant, H. (2014). Linking perception, cognition, and action: Psychophysical observations and neural network modelling. *PLoS One, 9*(7), e102553. doi:10.1371/journal.pone.0102553.
32. Ridderinkhof, K. R. (2014). Neurocognitive mechanisms of perception-action coordination: A review and theoretical integration. *Neuroscience & Biobehavioral Reviews, 46*, 3–29. doi:10.1016/j.neubiorev.2014.05.008.
33. Denckla, M. B. (1996). A theory and model of executive function: A neuropsychological perspective. In G. R. Lyon & N. A. Krasnegor (Eds.), *Attention, memory, and executive function* (pp. 263–278). Baltimore, MD: Paul H. Brookes.
34. Osterrieth, P. (1944). Le test de copie d'une figure complexe. *Archieves de Psychologie, 30*, 206–356.
35. Shorr, J. S., Delis, D. C., & Massman, P. J. (1992). Memory for the Rey-Osterrieth figure: Perceptual clustering, encoding, and storage. *Neuropsychology, 6*, 43–50.
36. Weber, R., Riccio, C., & Cohen, M. (2013). Does Rey complex figure copy performance measure executive function in children? *Applied Neuropsychology: Child, 2*, 6–12.
37. Darki, F., & Klingberg, T. (2015). The role of fronto-parietal and fronto-striatal networks in the development of working memory: A longitudinal study. *Cerebral Cortex, 25*(6), 1587–1595.
38. Cole, M. W., Reynolds, J. R., Power, J. D., Repovs, G., Anticevic, A., & Braver, T. S. (2013). Multi-task connectivity reveals flexible hubs for adaptive task control. *Nature Neuroscience, 16*, 1348–1355.
39. Cisek, P., & Pastor-Bernier, A. (2014). On the challenges and mechanisms of embodied decisions. *Philosophical Transactions of the Royal Society: Series B. Biological Sciences, 369*(1655), 20130479. doi:10.1098/rstb.2013.0479.
40. Bryan, K. L., & Hale, J. B. (2001). Differential effects of left and right cerebral vascular accidents on language competency. *Journal of the International Neuropsychological Society, 7*, 655–664.

41. Vakalopoulos, C. (2013). The developmental basis of visuomotor capabilities and the causal nature of motor clumsiness to cognitive and empathetic dysfunction. *Cerebellum, 12*(2), 212–223.
42. Mann, V. (1998). Language problems: A key to early reading problems. In B. Wong (Ed.), *Learning about learning disabilities* (pp. 213–228). Orlando, FL: Academic Press.
43. Miller, C. J., Sanchez, J., & Hynd, G. W. (2003). Neurological correlates of reading disabilities. In L. Swanson & S. Graham (Eds.), *Handbook of research on learning disabilities* (pp. 242–255). New York, NY: Guilford Press.
44. Geary, D. C. (2013). Learning disabilities in mathematics: Recent advances. In H. L. Swanson, K. Harris, & S. Graham (Eds.), *Handbook of learning disabilities* (2nd ed., pp. 239–255). New York, NY: Guilford Press.
45. Kaufmann, L., Mazzocco, M. M., Dowker, A., von Aster, M., Göbel, S. M., Grabner, R. H., ... Nuerk, H.-C. (2013). Dyscalculia from a developmental and differential perspective. *Frontiers in Psychology, 4*, 516. doi:10.3389/fpsyg.2013.00516.
46. Feifer, S. G., & Della Toffalo, D. A. (2005). *The neuropsychology of mathematics: Diagnosis and intervention*. Middletown, MD: School Neuropsych Press.
47. Voogd, J., Schraa-Tam, C. K. L., van der Geest, J. N., & De Zeeuw, C. I. (2010). Visuomotor cerebellum in human and nonhuman primates. *Cerebellum, 11*(2), 392–410.
48. Cortese, S., Kelly, C., Chabernaud, C., Proal, E., Di Martino, A., Milham, M. P., & Castellanos, F. X. (2012). Toward systems neuroscience of ADHD: A meta-analysis of 55 fMRI studies. *American Journal of Psychiatry, 169*, 1038–1055.
49. Koziol, L. F., Budding, D. E., & Chidekel, D. (2013). *ADHD as a model of brain-behavior relationships*. New York, NY: Springer.
50. Koziol, L. F. (2014). *The myth of executive functioning: Missing elements in conceptualization, evaluation, and assessment*. New York, NY: Springer.

Chapter 7
Summary

"I never think of the future. It comes soon enough."

Albert Einstein

"The time to repair the roof is when the sun is shining."

John F. Kennedy

"You Can't Teach an Old Dog New Tricks": Where Did Clinical Neuropsychology Go Wrong?

Many people are taught that when writing a manuscript, it is useful to apply three organizational principles. First, an introduction should describe what the text of the article or the subsequent chapters of the book are about. Second, the remaining text should expand upon that basic structure. Third, the summary should reiterate the basic "bullet points" that were presented in the preceding sections. In other words, the writer(s) should initially focus upon what he/she will be writing about or presenting. Then, the substantive information should be written. Finally, the summary should tell the reader about what was just previously presented. One of the co-authors of this series once attended a conference where the presenter stated: "first I tell them what I'm going to say; then I say it. Then I tell them what I spoke about." In ending this manuscript, we are essentially following that simple organizational framework, with an occasional deviation for the purpose of integration. At the end, what might be termed an "epilogue" is presented, but in this case, it is more of a summary of a summary.

Clinical neuropsychological assessment has traditionally been based upon a cortico-centric perspective which considers most behaviors are driven by conscious cognitive control. *ADHD as a Model of Brain-Behavior Relationships* [10] and *The Myth of Executive Functioning* [11] described how cognition, and behavior, are the products of interactions between the *vertically organized,* cortico-striatal and cerebro-cerebellar systems. Within this view, the primary focus of cognition is upon

© Springer International Publishing Switzerland 2016

L.F. Koziol et al., *Large-Scale Brain Systems and Neuropsychological Testing,*
DOI 10.1007/978-3-319-28222-0_7

action control. Cortico-centric models consider cognition as static. However, the cortico-striatal and cerebro-cerebellar models view cognition and behavior as dynamic, since people are always in constant interaction with a changing environment [1]. This requires movement, and within this dynamic model, the primary purpose of cognition in action control. Cognition, both explicitly and implicitly, links perceptions and ideas with the appropriate actions in order to adapt within this interactive paradigm. There really are no commercially available neuropsychological tests that are interpreted in a way that is consistent with this paradigm. Furthermore, advances within various branches of the neurosciences reveal that all cognition and behaviors are the product of dynamically changing patterns of functional connectivity that occur between large scale brain systems, or networks [2–7]. While neuropsychological assessment has been criticized from a variety of viewpoints, one of the biggest criticisms is its poor localization properties. Although we can argue that neuropsychological tests are reliable samples of cognition when considered from a "static" functional viewpoint, their localization properties are poor because all cognition, and behavior, are the manifestation of brain system interactions which are both localized and distributed, a process which neuropsychological tests were never intended to measure. From a historical perspective, the "static" view of neuropsychology has also focused on quantification. However, how can interactive processes be reduced to numbers for the purpose of artificial quantification when they do not align with either neural brain network interactions or practical day-to-day behaviors?

The current volume is a treatise on clinical neuropsychological test interpretation. We did not eliminate the quantification inherent in the scoring and interpretation of certain neuropsychological tests. However, we did closely examine the assumptions and properties of the statistical "normal distribution." We identified certain skills that can be interpreted within that framework, as well as those properties of cognition and behavior that cannot be interpreted within the confines and limitations of what has been traditionally been termed "the Bell-shaped curve." We noted that certain tests and procedures are "forced" to artificially meet the assumptions of the normal distribution. We have asked the practitioner to view certain cognitive functions in a completely different way and to interpret data from different perspectives. This approach hopefully takes the clinician a step away from overly simplistic quantification which does not contribute to understanding of the patient.

We also reviewed the interpretative strategy of test score comparisons. We applied this paradigm to the interpretation of learning and memory tests, resurrecting a paradigm proposed by Reitan and Davison [8], in which the individual subject acts as his or her own "control," rather than comparing a test score to a "normative sample" which results in an interpretation that is frequently misleading. It was demonstrated that by comparing *relevant test scores* to each other, a considerable amount of information can be derived. In fact, the interpretation that emerges becomes synergistic because it generates information that would never be known by interpreting any single test in isolation. We also stressed that this methodology requires considerable knowledge and skill about how tests are constructed, and how these tests are driven by the relevant underlying neuro-anatomical substrates.

In order to try to make a neuropsychological evaluation a more diagnostically powerful product, we examined the concept of "pathognomonic signs." These are behavioral signs that point to neuropsychological pathology in each and every instance. These types of behaviors are well known in certain disease processes. However, these potential pathognomonic signs of pathology have not been well studied in pediatric, neuro-developmental populations. Therefore, we proposed several pathognomonic signs observed in cases of neurodevelopmental pathologies. We stressed how test publishers often "force" or transform these signs, which follow a *dichotomous distribution*, into the normal distribution of a bell-shaped curve. We described how this process of statistical transformation might significantly reduce the risk of making a false positive error, while at the same time, mask or "hide" a symptom of pathology. During this discussion, it was also emphasized that the burden of knowledge and understanding is incumbent upon the clinical practitioner, since tests, and symptoms which the tests purport to measure, are simply not all equivalent. Attempting to view these different test paradigms as measuring the same processes, even though the "names" of certain behaviors might be identical, will almost always result in interpretative error. We discussed how it is extremely important to have considerable information about how any test is constructed, along with a comprehensive understanding of the neuro-biologic substrates that support accurate and inaccurate performance, for proper test interpretation. We also included a chapter on taking a relevant history, and we demonstrated how various aspects of a developmental history might increase the likelihood of a neurodevelopmental disorder. In this way, we were able to separate the concept of "at risk" factors from the pathology that is always inherent when using the terminology of specific or "pathognomonic signs." Identifying a risk factor from any individual's history does not necessarily equate to a later onset developmental disorder; but the term pathognomonic literally identifies a symptom of pathology that typically assists in leading to a greater understanding of the individual's functioning, if not increasing the likelihood of a given diagnosis. Therefore, to practice clinical neuropsychological assessment in this century, the practitioner needs an extensive and current knowledge base, as well as a strong experiential background.

As previously noted, today's knowledge of brain-behavior relationships includes an understanding of large scale brain networks and how these systems interact for the completion of any given task. In this regard, the final chapter had two purposes of equal importance. First, we made an attempt, whenever this was appropriate, to identify the various brain networks that are likely recruited during the performance of certain commonly known and used neuropsychological tests. We hope that our discussion took the reader at least one step closer to "currency" for the application of these tests within the framework of large scale brain systems. The field of clinical neuropsychological evaluation has a bit of "catching-up" to do, and our goal was to move in that direction. The simplistic viewpoint of cognition as a static entity no longer has meaningful application for the way in which behavior is organized within the brain. Primate and human brains are characterized by large scale brain systems, and patterns of functional connectivity within and between these systems represent our current understanding of brain-behavior relationships, in sickness and health.

Second, another purpose of our final chapter was to illustrate how current, commonly available neuropsychological tests can be administered in a slightly different way to provide the examiner with enriched interpretative information. In a nutshell, we attempted to demonstrate how tests might be utilized and interpreted within an "interactive" paradigm. As reviewed in *The Myth of Executive Functioning* [8], people generally function on "automatic pilot." Automatic behaviors are adaptive behaviors that must be learned. We proposed that "practice effect" need not be avoided, dependent upon the task in question. When tasks, or behaviors, are acquired, they become independent of cognitive control [9]. We attempted to demonstrate how different task administrations can assess this process, but because of space limitations, our focus was on the functions of the cerebellum, two of which are error detection and correction in order to achieve automaticity. In other examples, we attempted to demonstrate the process of perception-action coupling, a dynamic aspect of working memory, and how this can be literally "trained" for specific tasks. Similarly, we illustrated by prediction the behaviors that are exhibited when this type of linkage does not occur. We hope this discussion stimulated the reader's thinking to allow he or she to formally develop modifications in test administration more consistent with current conceptualizations of brain-behavior relationships.

We believe that this volume and the previously mentioned volumes [10, 11] provide the reader with new information about the vertically organized brain, and practical recommendations how to put this knowledge into clinical practice. It is recognized different readers possess different levels of knowledge and experience. These factors are critical variables because they provide the underpinning for the degree to which these volumes will be useful. While we have sought to make our case examples instructive, we never intended for anyone who reads this current volume to be "convinced" of anything. That goal would be terribly unrealistic. By analogy, any adult person who becomes fluent in a foreign language will almost always see that language differently from native speakers. Every author who participated in the writing of this book was originally trained in a cortico-centric model of cognition. However, after a number of years in clinical practice, we started to realize that certain tests and procedures we administered just didn't "make sense." All of us attempted to stay current in our knowledge base, but not necessarily by restricting ourselves to neuropsychology journals. Instead, we read journal articles from the field of cognitive science; from cognitive neuroscience; from the field of functional neuroimaging; from the fields of occupational therapy and neuropsychiatry, and even from anthropology. Gradually, we drifted away from the traditional field of neuropsychology we were initially trained in. In a sense, we were analogous to the adult becoming fluent in a foreign language. We will never understand as deeply as the "experts" within the fields from which we acquired information. However, we are conversant, or reasonably fluent, in each of these fields, and given the fact we are all experienced in neuropsychology, we believe we were capable of taking "the best from all worlds" in order to present the ideas in this volume in an understandable, practical way. If we have helped just one practitioner move forward in developing their knowledge about how they think about patients, we have achieved our goal.

There is much, much more work to be done. But this work is incumbent upon other practitioners to help move the field forward.

What does any of this have to do with the commonly known saying, "you can't teach an old dog new tricks?" Absolutely nothing! Traditional (i.e., cortico-centric) clinical neuropsychology might be considered an "old dog." After all, the field has been around for a long time. We didn't present any "new tricks." In fact, we did not even present any new ideas! Therefore, what is the point? We wrote this treatise based on information that has been known for a very long time about the vertically organized brain. We "fleshed out" or expanded upon known ideas using information gleaned from recent advances in our knowledge of subcortical processes and brain networks. We are baffled that the field, and its clinical practitioners, have not applied any of this historic information to current clinical neuropsychological assessment practices. The list of contributors to the history of clinical neuropsychological assessment is quite impressive. Yet somehow things went "wrong" for the field because important ideas were left behind, and inconvenient truths ignored. For some reason, many practitioners have seemed content in relying upon intuition, misinformed "logic," and tradition.

For example, consider the following quotes:

> "... performance on any given test is multi-determined, and for this reason, it is not always possible to posit a single explanation for any given response. Nevertheless, of the many potential factors that may have to be taken into account, success and failure on a given task are most often found to depend upon the degree to which a subject possesses or lacks the ability or abilities implicit in or required by the task. This presupposes that one knows what a test measures or purports to measure. Our knowledge in this respect still leaves much to be desired...." ([12], p. 482).

> "... any scores representing sums or averages of disparate data obtained from tests of brain functions and mental abilities—can obscure specific facets of a subject's neuropsychological status or misrepresent it generally." ([13], p. 351).

In our view, these are extremely powerful quotations because they are both history and fact. Nobody would question the credentials of these individuals. Matarazzo is saying that tests should not be interpreted unless the practitioner understands the cognitive processes that support test performance. He reminds us that tests used in cognitive assessment cannot be interpreted according to face validity. Similarly, he is explicitly stating that testing tasks require certain abilities that are implicit, and that these implicit cognitions need to be investigated and understood. We hope this sounds familiar because the exact same points were made in previous chapters. We included the neuroscientific principles that support Matarazzo's position. We described how certain explicit tasks can become implicitly automatic by capitalizing upon the potential benefits of "practice effect."

Lezak wrote about how combining test scores generate a quotient that literally hides the skills and capacities we are trying to measure. This was also addressed in our text. In these ways, we are genuinely puzzled about what went wrong in the practice of clinical neuropsychology, a field which has been stagnant for over 40 years.

With respect to tradition in the practice of neuropsychology, Kent [14] summed-up the current state of affairs very succinctly by stating,

> "...it is assumed the Wechsler Memory Scale is ecologically valid, since it has been in clinical use since 1940 [15], and therefore has passed the test of time, despite reports of individuals who perform normally on it yet still demonstrate extreme forgetfulness in normal daily activities [16]. As an example of the gap between what a test purports to measure, and what it actually measures, one need look no further than the most current version of the Wechsler Memory Scale. It was specifically designed to measure auditory and visual immediate and delayed memory, and visual working memory. The authors of the technical manual [17], however, acknowledge that factor analysis does not support the immediate and delayed distinction. Despite this, clinicians regularly refer to differences in immediate and delayed memory in their reports, likely due to "customary professional practices" and not having read the technical manual. The continued use of the WMS to assess immediate and delayed memory is just one glaring example of the lack of evidence- or theory-based practice among psychologists and neuropsychologists."

Where did neuropsychology go wrong? Does it really matter? Perhaps things went wrong because practitioners never really had control over the tools they use to begin with? No. This is a lame excuse. For example, neuropsychologists like Reitan and Luria did not have organizations or test publishers that offered an array of tests for purchase; they designed testing procedures. If individuals without much of an organized knowledge base were able to construct evaluation tasks, it seems logical to think that in this day and age, with a voluminous scientific knowledge base, a profession with a huge membership that refers to itself as clinical neuropsychology should be capable of updating testing tasks and constructing new ones. Perhaps the field shirked its responsibility by taking things for granted. Trying to answer these questions is a waste of time. It doesn't really matter because in the present, we can only look back on history, understand what is going on within the field presently, use this information, and accept that it is the responsibility of practitioners to move the field forward. If the field simply waits, we might expect that in the next 40 years, the field will be in the same position it is in right now. If the field remains complacent, we can envision universities offering a course titled "The History of Neuroscience." In that course, neuropsychology will be portrayed as a dinosaur, an example of how brain-behavior relationships used to be studied with a methodology that has become extinct.

References

1. Cisek, P., & Kalaska, J. F. (2010). Neural mechanisms for interacting with a world full of action choices. *Annual Review of Neuroscience, 33*, 269-298.
2. Castellanos, F. X., & Proal, E. (2012). Large-scale brain systems in ADHD: beyond the prefrontal-striatal model. *Trends in Cognitive Sciences, 16*(1), 17-26.
3. Yeo, B. T., Krienen, F. M., Sepulcre, J., Sabuncu, M. R., Lashkari, D., Hollinshead, M., . . . Buckner, R. L. (2011). The organization of the human cerebral cortex estimated by intrinsic functional connectivity. *Journal of Neurophysiology, 106*(3), 1125-1165.
4. Koziol, L. F., Barker, L. A., Joyce, A. W., & Hrin, S. (2014). Structure and function of large-scale brain systems. *Applied Neuropsychology: Child, 3*(4), 236-244.

5. Koziol, L. F., Barker, L. A., Joyce, A. W., & Hrin, S. (2014). The small-world organization of large-scale brain systems and relationships with subcortical structures. *Applied Neuropsychology: Child, 3*(4), 245-252.
6. Koziol, L. F., Barker, L. A., Joyce, A. W., & Hrin, S. (2014). Large-scale brain systems and subcortical relationships: The vertically organized brain. *Applied Neuropsychology: Child, 3*(4), 253-263.
7. Koziol, L. F., Barker, L. A., Hrin, S., &Joyce, A. W. (2014). Large-scale brain systems and subcortical relationships: Practical applications. *Applied Neuropsychology: Child, 3*(4), 264-273.
8. Reitan, R. M. & Davison, L. A. (1974). *Clinical neuropsychology: Current applications.* Washington, DC: Hemisphere Publishing Corp.
9. Ito, M. (2012). *The cerebellum: Brain for an implicit self.* Upper Saddle River, NJ: FT Press.
10. Koziol, L. F., Budding, D. E., & Chidekel, D. (2013). *ADHD as a model of brain-behavior relationships.* New York, NY: Springer.
11. Koziol, L. F. (2014). *The myth of executive functioning: Missing elements in conceptualization, evaluation, and assessment.* New York, NY: Springer.
12. Matarazzo, J. D. (1972). *Wechsler's measurement and appraisal of adult intelligence* (5th and enlarged ed.). Baltimore, MD: Lippincott Williams & Wilkins.
13. Lezak, M. D. (1988). IQ: R.I.P. *Journal of Clinical and Experimental Neuropsychology, 10,* 351–361.
14. Kent, P. L. (2015). Working memory: A selective review. *Applied Neuropsychology: Child.* Retrieved from 22 Aug 2015.
15. Wechsler, D. (1945). A standardized memory scale for clinical use. *The Journal of Psychology, 19,* pp. 87–95.
16. Heilman, K., & Valenstein, E. (2003). *Clinical neuropsychological assessment* (4th ed.). New York, NY: Oxford University Press.
17. Holdnack, J. A., & Drozdick, L. W. (2009). *WMS-IV technical and interpretive manual.* San Antonio, TX: Pearson.
18. Lezak, M. D., Howieson, D. B., Bigler, E. D., & Tranel, D. (2012). Neuropsychological assessment (5th ed.). New York, NY: Oxford University Press.

Index

B
Bell-shaped curve, 130
  basal ganglia, 73
  chance variation and statistical vs. clinical
      significance, 56–58
  clinician's knowledge base, 71
  cognitive processes, 72
  frontal lobe functions, 74
  frontal lobe subtest, 72
  functional neuroanatomy, 71
  interim, 71
  intra-individual and test score comparisons,
      63–65
  level of performance methodology, 71
  neuroanatomical concepts, 73
  neuropsychological tests, 49, 50, 71
  problem-solving, 74
  statistical conversions vs. normal
      distributions, 58–60
  statistical processes, 54–56
  test interpretation, 49
  testing and evaluation process, 50
  Tower of London test, 73–75
  treatment planning, 75
  WCST, 72, 75
Brain-behavior relationships, 131
Bullet points, 129

C
California Verbal Learning Test, 2nd Edition
      (CVLT II), 63, 69
Cerebellum, 132
Cerebro-cerebellar systems, 129
Clinical neuropsychological assessment, 129, 130

Cognitive assessment, 133
Continuous performance tests (CPTs), 84–85
Cortico-centric model, 130, 132

D
Default mode network (DMN), 88, 114
Dorsal attention network (DAN), 106

F
Frontal-parietal network (FPN), 87

G
Gomez-Lopez-Hernandez Syndrome, 90
Gordon Diagnostic System, 87

I
"Intact" phonological processing, 59

M
Medial temporal lobe memory system
  Alzheimer's disease, 68
  anterior brain system, 70
  characteristics, 65
  CVLT, 67
  CVLT-II, 69
  depression, 68
  "False Positive" errors, 67
  frontal-striatal systems, 70
  learning and memory tasks, 66
  memory evaluation, 67

© Springer International Publishing Switzerland 2016
L.F. Koziol et al., *Large-Scale Brain Systems and Neuropsychological Testing*,
DOI 10.1007/978-3-319-28222-0

Medial temporal lobe memory system (*cont.*)
  MTL system, 66
  neuro-biologic substrate, 65
  "non-verbal" learning/memory tests, 66
  normal distribution, 66
  raw score data, 68, 69
  RCFT, 68
  recognition memory system, 65
  Rey Complex Figure Test, 70
  Weschler Memory Scale, 69
  WMS-IV, 68, 70
  z-score, 67
Mild cognitive impairment (MCI), 82
Mirsky model of attention, 87

N
Neurocognitive processes, 59
Neurodevelopmental disorder, 83–84, 131
Neurodevelopmental pathology, 5–8, 10–20
  ADHD, 5–9
    "at risk" factors, 8
    Apgar Scores, 10
    ATNR, 16, 17
    *Attention, Balance and Coordination:
      The A.B.C.'s of Learning Success*, 16
    automatic crawling, 19
    axiom, 8
    developmental history data, 20
    diagnosis, 6
    dorsal attention network, 18
    feeding, language and reward, 12–14
    guiding children's learning, 7
    hyperbilirubinemia, 14, 15
    like symptoms, 3
    neurodevelopment, 7
    neuropsychological evaluation, 5
    premature birth, 11, 12
    prenatal reflexes, 15
    STNR, 18
    testing, 7
  birth complications, 4
  clinical neuropsychological interview and
      evaluation, 3
  disorders, 22
  erroneous and misleading history, 20, 21
  factors, 1
  hypotonia, 22
  integration, 3
  motor and neurocognitive functions, 5
  psychostimulant medication, 4
  recommendations, 3
  risk factors, 2
  second opinion, 22

  speech/language pathology and
      occupational therapy, 1
  symptoms, 3
  testing, 22
  treatment plans, 4
Neurodevelopmental skill, 60
Neuropsychological assessment, 60
Neuropsychological evaluation, 103–109
  adaptive behaviors, 102
  ADHD, 114, 122
  automatic/routine level, 103
  basal ganglia, 103
  brain function, 102, 123
  brain-behavior relationships, 103
  cerebellar abnormalities, 111
  cerebellar circuitry system, 103
  cerebellar tonsils, 109
  cerebellar vermis, 109
  cerebellum, 103
  clinical information, 115
  cognitive referencing, 111
  conscious cognitive control, 101
  cortex and cerebellum function, 111
  DAN network, 111
  deficiencies, 101
  demonstration approach, 115
  demonstration methodology, 114
  DMN, 114
  examiner-directed approach, 102
  executive function, 118
  FPN and SMN, 118
  geometry, 121
  Gomez-Lopez-Hernandez Syndrome, 109
  hemisphere, 121
  immediate memory trial, 112
  instruments, 103
  interpretation, 101, 114
  lack of integrity, brain systems, 114, 119
  linkage system, 114
  measures, 102
  MRI findings, cerebellar hemispheres,
      109–111
  novelty-routinization principle, 102
  perceive-think-respond methodology, 102
  perception-action coupling, 112, 113
  practice effect
    administration protocol, 108
    bilateral medial temporal lobe
        resection, 106
    brain takes, 104
    brain-behavior relationships, 104
    cerebellum, 107, 108
    cerebro-cerebellar interactions, 107
    cognitive tests, 104

cognitive/motor sequences, 107
conscious awareness, 105
conscious control, 108
consecutive trials, 107
coupling, 108
DAN, 106
declarative memory system and
    procedural learning system, 106
FPN, 106–107
implicit learning, 107, 109
interpretation, 109
learning, 103, 105
The *learning and memory of
    procedures*, 104
logical intuition informs, 105
mental tracking, 108
procedural and implicit learning, 105
processing speed, 109
sensory-motor network, 106
stimulus-based characteristics, 105
TMT, 106
true ability, 104
VAN, 106
WCST, 104
working memory component, 108
working memory functions, 107
problem-solving, 102
products, 114
RCFT performance, 115
Rey-Osterreith Complex Figure Test, 112
romboencephalitis, 109
serial-order processing methodology, 102
test administration, 113
traditional verbal versus visual-spatial
    dichotomy, 121
VAN and DAN, 118
ventral and dorsal attention networks, 103
verbal *vs.* non-verbal dichotomy, 102
visual field search strategy, 111
visual network, 123
visual-motor, 112, 121
visual-spatial deficit, 113, 114
visual-spatial functioning, 103
visual-spatial skills, 121
Wechsler scales, 102
working memory, 118
Neuropsychological test, 31–36, 39, 40
    analysis, sensory and motor data, 41–44
    brain function standardization, 28
    categories, 28
    challenges, 45–46
    clinical data
        allergies and autism, 35
        anoxic brain injury, 34

auditory attention, 31
brain injury, 35
clinical judgment, 34
construction and performance, 32
cultural factors, 33
executive function, 31
frontal lobe tests, 31
fronto-parietal network (FPN), 31
neural processing, 32
ongoing interactions, 32
outcomes, 35
revision and recency, 33
severe emotional reaction, 34
sinus, 35
validity, 31
Wechsler Intelligence Scales, 31
Wisconsin Card Sort Test, 31
clinical evaluation, 29
computerized test programs, 28, 29
differentiation, 29
distribution, cognitive functions and
    behaviors, 28
fact, 30
interpret data, 30, 45
interpretation, 27
level of performance, 38–39
levels of inference, 37–38
measures, 28
neuro-biologic substrate, 30
pathognomonic signs, 41
pattern analysis
    language, 39
    letter or phonemic fluency, 40
    semantic classification system, 39
    symptom identification, 40
    synergistic, 39
performances, 29
practitioner's knowledge of
    neuroanatomy, 30
quantification, behavior (*see* Quantification
    of behavior)
RDoC methodology, 29
reports, 27
sensory and motor data, 42–44
symptoms or pathology, 29, 30
transformation, 28
Neuropsychology, 132, 134
Normal distribution, 130
    accelerated or robust acquisition, 52
    bell shaped curve, 51
    cognitive/behavioral functions, 52
    "IQ", 50
    limitations, 52–54
    standard deviation, 51

Normal distribution (*cont.*)
    standard score, 51
    statistical principles, 50
    symmetry, 50

P
Pathognomonic signs, 41, 131
    adult pathologies, 81
    alerting/anticipatory stimuli, 86
    ambiguity, 84
    aphasia and agnosia, 82
    behaviors, 79
    borderline statistical category, 89
    brain structures and neural networks, 87
    brain-behavior relationships, 85
    cerebellar control model, 81
    cerebellum, 90
    child's reading development, 92
    clinical neuropsychology, 79
    cognitive and academic psychology, 86
    CPTs, stop signal tasks and go-no go
        paradigms, 86–88
    decision making points, 96
    diagnosis, ADHD, 84, 89
    dichotomous distribution, 79
    disinhibition, 88
    disorientation, 81
    distractibility, 91
    DMN, 88
    "double deficit" hypothesis, 93
    DSM, 85
    dysfunction, 80
    dyslexia, 92
    errors of commission, 90
    errors of omission, 90
    executive functioning, 91
    false positive and negative errors,
        82, 94
    finger-to-nose test, 80, 81
    FPN, 88, 93
    frontal inhibition, 87
    frontal-striatal and the cerebro-cerebellar
        systems, 91
    interpretation, 80
    intuitive judgment, 80
    language-based skill, 91
    litmus test, 85
    Mirsky model of attention, 87
    motor skill, 92
    neuro-developmental disorders, 83–84

    novelty detector, 88
    oromotor control, 92
    phoneme awareness, 93
    phonological awareness, 93
    phonological processing, 80
    reading disorder, 95, 96
    school-aged children, 92
    speed-accuracy trade-off, 95
    sustained performance, 86
    test/battery of tests, 85
    TOVA, 85
    troubled waters, 84
    "umbrella-like" categorization, 80
    Vigilance Task of the GDS, 89
    "whole words", 94
Phonological processing, 58

Q
Quantification of behavior
    Arithmetic and Digit Span (DS) tests, 37
    conversion process, 36
    interpretive value, 36
    qualitative review, 37
    statistical normative standard, 36
    Wechsler Scales, 36
    WMI, 37

R
RCFT. *See* Rey Complex Figure Test
        (RCFT)
Recognition memory system, 65
Rey Complex Figure Test (RCFT),
        68, 112

S
Sensory and motor data, 42, 43
    bilateral motor programming, 42
    control, 42
    fingertip tapping, 43
    HRB, 41
    identification, 41
    integrative functions, 43
    limitations, 44
    NEPSY, 42, 43
    neuropsychological assessments, 42
    pincer finger grasp, 44
    programs, 44
    sequencing tasks, 44

T
Test of Variables of Attention (TOVA), 85
TMT. *See* Trail Making Tests (TMT)
Trail Making Tests (TMT), 106

V
VAN. *See* Ventral attention network (VAN)
Ventral attention network (VAN), 106
Visual acuity, 59

W
WCST. *See* Wisconsin Card Sorting Test
    (WCST)
Wechsler Memory Scale, 4th Edition
    (WMS-IV), 68
Wechsler Working Memory Index
    (WMI), 37
Wisconsin Card Sorting Test (WCST),
    72, 104

Printed in Great Britain
by Amazon

20756036R00095